PANIC
NATION

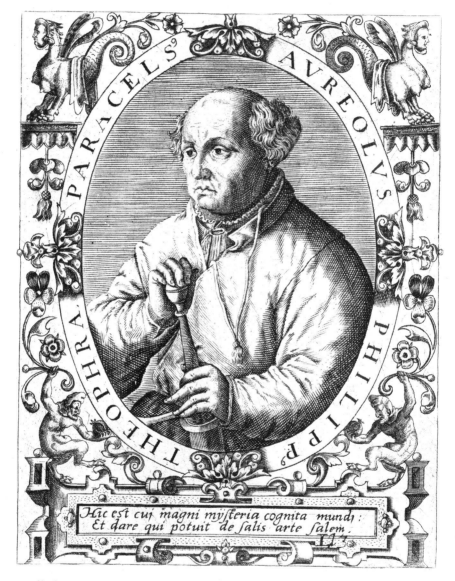

'All things are poison and nothing is without poison. It is the dose
that makes a thing poisonous.'

PERACELSUS, FATHER OF MODERN TOXICOLOGY, (1493-1541)

PANIC NATION

UNPICKING THE MYTHS WE'RE TOLD ABOUT FOOD AND HEALTH

EDITED BY STANLEY FELDMAN AND VINCENT MARKS

JOHN BLAKE

Published by John Blake Publishing Ltd,
3, Bramber Court, 2 Bramber Road,
London W14 9PB, England

www.blake.co.uk

First published in paperback in 2005

ISBN 1 84454 122 3

British Library Cataloguing-in-Publication Data: a catalogue record for
this book is available from the British Library.

Design by www.envydesign.co.uk

Printed in Great Britain by CPD, Wales

1 3 5 7 9 10 8 6 4 2

Papers used by John Blake Publishing are natural, recyclable products
made from wood grown in sustainable forests. The manufacturing
processes conform to the environmental regulations of the country of
origin.

Every attempt has been made to contact the relevant copyright-holders,
but some were unobtainable. We would be grateful if the appropriate
people could contact us.

Frontispiece © Wellcome

Dedicated to Carole and Averil for their patience,
understanding and love.

ACKNOWLEDGEMENTS

A glance at the list of distinguished contributors will reveal that this book is very much a joint effort, indeed, without the enthusiastic support of these experts the work would not carry as much authority as it does. We are indebted to the members of the Millennium Society who have helped us in identifying topics that they felt needed to be covered in the book. The views expressed are those of the authors and do not necessarily reflect the views of the editors or other contributors.

Scientists are used to communicating with each other in a genre that is often difficult for those outside their circle to understand. We are indebted to Jennie Bristow for her careful editing of the manuscripts so as to reduce any technical jargon to a minimum and to ensure that all the contributions are presented in a uniform, readily understable style.

We are grateful for the assistance and encouragement of John Blake, the publisher of this book and to James Ravenscroft who has helped nurse the book from its conception to its production. Finally, we are would like to acknowledge the advice and criticisms of our wives, and of the panel of 'guinea pig' readers, especially those on board the yacht *Holiday V11*.

EDITORS

Stanley Feldman gave up his biochemistry thesis on the metabolism of the woodlouse to study medicine in 1950. Qualified (hons) Westminster Medical School 1955. He trained as an anaesthetist at Westminster Hospital, Research Fellow at University Washington USA 1957–58. Senior Lecturer Postgraduate Medical School, 1962. Adviser in Post-Graduate Studies Faculty Anaesthetist 1965–70. Visiting Professor Stanford University USA 1967–68. Higginbotham Lecturer Dallas, Frederickson Orator Emory. Member Senate University London, Chair of Anaesthesia University London at Charing Cross and Westminster Medical Schools (later Imperial College School Medicine). Research adviser Royal National Orthopaedic Hospital 1994–97. Examiner in physiology for Faculty Anaesthetists, College of Surgeons and Dental Faculty.

Author/Editor of 12 textbooks on anaesthesia, including *Scientific Foundations of Anaesthesia, Mechanism of Action of Drugs* and *Drugs in Anaesthesia*. Editor *Journal Anaesthetic Pharmacology Review*. Contributor *Encyclopaedia Britannica*.

He has published over 100 peer-reviewed papers on molecular mechanisms of drug action and post-graduate education. His most recent publication is *Poison Arrows* (Metro Publishing), 2005.

The author of several textbooks, **Vincent Marks** went from Tottenham County School on a State Scholarship in 1948 to read medicine at Oxford. Since 1970, he has been Professor, now Emeritus, of Clinical Biochemistry at the University of Surrey in Guildford. Known internationally for his research on hypoglycaemia and diabetes, he has appeared as an expert witness in some of the world's most famous trials such as those of Claus von Bulow in America, Beverley Allitt in England and Colin Bouwer in New Zealand. His work on intestinal hormones led him to designate GIP the obesity hormone and his description of muesli-belt nutrition established him as one of the country's best-known nutritionists. A former president of the Association of Clinical Biochemists and erstwhile vice president of the Royal College of Pathologists. Vincent was a founder member of HealthWatch. He is now semi-retired and lives in Haslemere with his wife Averil. Both their children are lawyers.

NOTES ON CONTRIBUTORS

Professor **Paul Aichroth** was a consultant orthopaedic surgeon at the Westminster, Chelsea & Westminster and the Westminster Children's Hospitals over many years. His private work was undertaken mainly at the Wellington Hospital where he was Director of the Knee Surgery Unit. He is now Visiting Professor in the Department of Surgery, Imperial College, and continues teaching there. He exercises regularly!

Michael Baum is Emeritus Professor of Surgery and Visiting Professor of Medical Humanities University College London.

He qualified in medicine in 1960 and trained as a surgeon. FRCS in 1965 and MS in 1972. Appointed to Chair of Surgery at Kings College London 1980. MD 1986. Appointed to Chair of Surgery at the Royal Marsden Hospital in 1990. Past chairman of the UK Cancer Research, breast sub-committee, past president of the British Oncological Society, Chairman of the Council of the National Institute of Medical Humanities and President of the 2002 European Breast Cancer Conference. Author of numerous research papers and reports on cancer of the breast.

Dr **David A Bender** has a BSc in Biochemistry (University of Birmingham) and a PhD from the University of London; since 1970, he has taught nutrition and biochemistry to medical students and general students. He is currently Sub-Dean (teaching) of the Royal Free Hospital and University College Medical School and a senior lecturer in the Department of Biochemistry of University College London. In addition to over 100 research publications in nutritional biochemistry, he has written 16 textbooks and contributed chapters to others. He is Editor-in-Chief of *Nutrition Research Reviews* and an Executive Editor of the *Journal of the Science of Food and Agriculture*.

Dr **Michael Fitzpatrick** has been a general practitioner in East London for the past twenty years. He has written on a wide range of medical and political subjects, including AIDS, addictions and health scares for both medical publications and the mainstream media. He writes columns in *The Lancet* and the *British Journal of General Practice* and is a regular contributor to the online magazine *spiked* (www.spiked-online.com). He has also appeared frequently on radio and television, and in 1997 produced a critical programme on 'parenting' for the BBC. His book *The Tyranny of Health: Doctors and the Regulation of Lifestyle* was published by Routledge in 2001. His critique of complementary medicine is included in *Alternative Medicine – Should We Swallow It?*, published by the Institute of Ideas/Hodder and Stoughton in 2002. His latest book, *MMR and Autism: What Parents Need To Know* (Routledge) was published in 2004.

Professor **Paul Grob** was a GP for 40 years in a large Surrey practice. He held the Chair of General Practice and Health Care Research at the University of Surrey and was involved in a number of large international research projects, both in the field of education, satellite-mediated learning and clinical practices. In 1970, he was one of the first regional advisers in general practice to be appointed by the British Postgraduate Medical Federation and later became Associate Dean with a responsibility for standards in general practice together with the ongoing education of young doctors. He has published widely and is currently working at the University of Surrey on a project to explore how doctors can effectively learn from their mistakes.

Maurice Hanssen's interest in additives began a long time before they were identified on the pack. As a director of a leading manufacturer of wines and foods, he questioned why they were using additives which seemed unnecessary and found equally good or better products could be made without using so many. Later he became a successful consultant on food and health.

Author of 28 books including the bestseller *E for Additives*, he has sold over two and a half million copies in all. As a Chambellan of the Ordre des Coteaux de Champagne and a Lauréat of the World Master Chefs Society, he believes that our food should be delicious, healthy and fun.

Professor **John Henry** followed a career in general medicine and clinical toxicology at Guy's and St Thomas' Hospitals. He was appointed to the Chair in Accident and Emergency Medicine at Imperial College School of Medicine in 1997 and made a Consultant at St Mary's Hospital London. He has researched and written widely, and his interests cover all forms of acute poisoning and the medical complications of illicit drugs.

Mick Hume is editor of the online magazine *spiked* (www.spiked-online.com) and a columnist for *The Times*.

Dr **Lakshman Karalliedde** graduated from the University of Colombo, Sri Lanka and did his post-graduate training in anaesthesia at the Westminster and Royal Northern Hospitals London. At the Faculty of Medicine, Peradeniya, Sri Lanka, he developed a special interest in organophosphorus insecticide poisoning and abuse for decades and described the 'Intermediate Syndrome' of organophosphate poisoning. He resigned his post in Sri Lanka as Head of the Department of Anaesthesiology to return to the UK where he served as Senior Lecturer in Anaesthetics at United Medical & Dental Schools of Guy's & St Thomas' before joining the Medical Toxicology Unit of the Guy's & St Thomas' NHS Trust where he has been a consultant toxicologist for the past seven years. He was lead editor of *Organophosphates & Health* (Imperial College Press) and *Handbook of Drug Interactions* (Hodder Arnold) and has published widely on organophosphate and pesticide poisoning, contributing to many textbooks including *Davidson's Principles & Practice of Medicine*.

Dr **Malcolm Kendrick** is a medical doctor who has spent many years researching the causes of heart disease. He designed and set up the educational website for the European Society of Cardiology (ESC) and worked closely with a number of International Medical Societies to develop a Europe-wide system of Continuing Medical Education. He also set up the first website for the National Institute of Clinical Excellence (NICE). Malcolm has written widely on heart disease and has been critical of the so-called 'cholesterol hypothesis' for many years. Some of his more provocative writing on the area can be found at the website of the International Network of Cholesterol Sceptics (www.thincs.org).

Sir **Peter Lachmann** is a medical immunologist. He is Emeritus Professor of Immunology in the University of Cambridge and a Fellow of Christ's College. He is also President of the Federation of European Academies of Medicine

He was the founder President of the UK Academy of Medical Sciences (1998–2002); Biological Secretary of the Royal Society (1993–98) and President of the Royal College of Pathologists (1990–93). He served on UNESCO's international bioethics committee from 1993–98.

For the Royal Society, he has chaired working groups on BSE and on GMOs.

Dr **James Le Fanu** is a general practitioner in South London and medical columnist of the *Sunday* and *Daily Telegraph*. He graduated from Cambridge University and the Royal London Hospital in 1974 and held junior hospital posts at Whipps Cross Hospital, the Royal Free, St Mary's and the Bristol Royal Infirmary. He has made original contributions to medical journals on many subjects including the threat of a heterosexual AIDS epidemic, passive smoking, poverty and health and the dietary causes of heart disease. His history of post-war medicine, *The Rise and Fall of Modem Medicine*, was published by Little, Brown in June 1999.

Dr **Sandy Macnair** qualified in medicine from St Andrews University and, after a stint in general practice, joined the pharmaceutical industry organising both fundamental and clinical research for several companies in Europe, Africa, Australasia and North America. Latterly, he has been an independent consultant to a number of primary food producers including those of sugar, eggs, milk and salt, with regard to their impact on the public health.

Sam Shuster is Emeritus Professor of Dermatology, University of Newcastle Upon Tyne and Honorary Consultant to the Department of Dermatology, Norfolk and Norwich University Hospital. He qualified in medicine at UCL, followed by a PhD in physiology, and, after junior clinical and research posts in the Royal Postgraduate School of Medicine, was appointed Lecturer in Medicine in the Welsh National School of Medicine. An interest in endocrinology and metabolism led on to dermatological research, and he started the Skin Research Unit in The Institute of Dermatology, and was subsequently appointed to the Chair of Dermatology in Newcastle, then the main centre for skin research in the UK. He was President of The European Society for Dermatological Research and a member of many academic and government committees. He has published many papers and books on clinical and fundamental dermatological research, including aging, UV radiation, and basic and clinical pharmacology; he has an interest in sports medicine.

Professor **John Studd** is a Consultant Gynaecologist, Chelsea and Westminster Hospital and also Professor of Gynaecology at Imperial College. He trained in Southern Rhodesia and Birmingham and has been a Consultant in Nottingham and King's College Hospital, London before moving to Chelsea and Westminster. He started the first HRT clinic in Europe and still has a considerable research output for HRT, menopausal symptoms, osteoporosis and premenstrual syndrome.

Lord Taverne – **Dick Taverne** QC – has been an influential voice in politics for many years. As a Labour MP, he become Financial Secretary to the Treasury; in 1973, he stood and was elected as an Independent Social Democrat and today he sits in the House of Lords as a Liberal Democrat. Recently his main interest has been science and society and three years ago he founded the charity Sense About Science to promote the evidence-based approach to scientific issues. He is the author of *The March of Unreason: Science, Democracy and the New Fundamentalism* published in 2005.

CONTENTS

PREFACE

BY STANLEY FELDMAN
AND VINCENT MARKS

'We ought to recourse to experimentation and not suffer ourselves to be deluded by unfounded theory or specious argument.'

ABBÉ FELICE FONTANA, 1775

This book is an attempt to set the record straight, to counter 'unfounded theory and specious argument'.

We have been through a period when a mixture of half-truths, tendentious beliefs and unsubstantiated opinions has been presented in the media as incontrovertible, scientifically proven facts. Many of these ideas have originated from overzealous pressure groups or presentations by special-interest lobbies. The more improbable the story, the more attention it receives from a press hungry for sensational news. The stories are seldom analysed, or their contents challenged by the scientific community. As a result, many of these ideas have become accepted – both by the public and by responsible official bodies who lack the knowledge or the political will to challenge them – as self-evident truths.

The idea for the book was born out of our frustration at the credence given to the avalanche of slanted, improbable and inaccurate scare stories that fuel what Mick Hume has described as 'an epidemic of epidemics'. The stories of which we complain are those that are presented as facts of the 'everybody knows' variety or reflect the opinions of certain self-promoting experts with axes to grind.

The frustration and anger at our impotence to counter this growing band of scare stories came to a head at a meeting of the Millennium Club in 2004. At this meeting, a group of senior academics interested in healthcare problems suggested that it was time to set the record straight. The idea of this book was to get a group of truly independent experts to examine the scientific evidence behind some of the current scare stories and to present it in a manner that would make it easily understandable by the general public. Our aim is to separate what is probably true about a given subject from that which is merely opinion. To this end we have sought contributions from scientists, academic doctors and independent journalists who have expertise in a given subject. We have asked them to present the facts behind these issues so that readers can determine for themselves where the truth lies. Each contribution represents the interpretation put on the facts by its author and does not necessarily reflect the collective opinion of the editors or other contributors. If we have succeeded in persuading the reader to think again about the 'unfounded theories and specious arguments' with which we are bombarded, it will have served part of its purpose of being an interesting, informative and enjoyable read.

INTRODUCTION: PANIC NATION

BY MICK HUME

Since the panic about a SARS epidemic gripped the world in 2003, the New Labour government's policy towards issues such as bioterrorism and SARS in the UK has been based on the principle of 'organised paranoia'. This memorable but little-known phrase was coined by Geoff Mulgan, former head of the powerful Downing Street Performance and Innovation Unit. Mulgan was speaking at a conference entitled 'Panic Attack: Interrogating our Obsession with Risk', organised by *spiked* – the online publication of which I am editor – at the Royal Institution in May 2003. He had a wry little smile on his face when he used those words, but he definitely was not joking.

Mulgan suggested that organised paranoia would help the government become better at spotting new risks such as SARS, BSE or bioterrorism 'before they become evident'. But how exactly do the seers and oracles of Whitehall hope to identify a potential risk before it has even become visible? By gazing into a crystal ball, perhaps?

Almost, it seems. The modern political equivalent of the crystal ball is the 'what if?' scenario, and this is increasingly becoming the stuff of policy-planning discussions on both sides of the Atlantic, especially post-9/11. It means that policy-makers dream up fantasy disasters (what if a terrorist infected with SARS crashed a petrol tanker into a nuclear power station?), and then try to plan how to deal with these hypothetical crises. Under the policy of organised paranoia, government and society are continually being re-educated to expect a worst-case scenario. This trend has the potential to become a real disaster for us all.

The advance of organised paranoia was what prompted *spiked* to organise the Panic Attack conference in the first place. It proved a timely event, taking place in the middle of the global SARS panic. The reaction to SARS became a powerful symbol of what is wrong. Here was a new but relatively minor epidemic that, in a sane society, would demand a serious response from the medical and epidemiological authorities. In our apparently less-than-sane society, however, officials from the World Health Organisation (WHO) downwards treated SARS as a cross between the black death and a bioterror attack, quarantining entire cities and damaging whole economies. Meanwhile, people across the world could be seen walking around wearing useless paper masks, a sort of modern equivalent of the medieval amulets used to ward off evil. The SARS panic turned into an outstanding example of the cure being worse than the disease, causing more damage in the real world than any fantastic 'what if?' scenario is likely to.

It is common to blame such outbreaks of irrationality on the supposed ignorance of 'ordinary people'. But Mulgan's remarks should serve to remind us that the suffocating, safety-first spirit of the age comes from the top down, that the precautionary principle has become a guiding light in public life. Major political, academic and scientific institutions now appear to be obsessed with risk and infected by the outlook of organised paranoia, with damaging consequences.

For instance, scary speculation about us all being doomed is traditionally associated with the crank forecasts of astrology. Yet it now seems to have crept into the science of astronomy, too. Martin

Rees, the UK's astronomer royal and a leading scientific figure, has published a major book entitled *Our Final Century: Will the Human Race Survive the Twenty-first Century?* In it, Rees argues that human civilisation has no more than a 50–50 chance of surviving the twenty-first century, because of the alleged 'dark side' of scientific and technological advance, and because our 'interconnected' world makes us more vulnerable to new risks. He advocates investment in space travel, not because we might want to push back the boundaries of exploration, but because we will need somewhere else to run to pretty soon, when we have destroyed the Earth. Not very long ago, this would have been rightly considered the stuff of science-fiction fantasies. Now it is put forward by a leading scientist, and taken seriously by many of his peers.

Not very long ago, the notion that the end of the world is nigh would have been the preserve of a few religious nutters marching up and down wearing sandwich boards. Now the astronomer royal offers it up for serious consideration. If this kind of stuff is allowed to go unchallenged, however, the end of the rational world may well be nigh.

The BBC, one of our leading national institutions, has become a particular champion of organised paranoia and the scaremongering 'what if?' scenario. Around the time of our Panic Attack conference, the BBC broadcast a TV docudrama entitled *The Day Britain Stopped*, about how a series of events supposedly brings the entire transport system crashing to a halt at the end of 2003, with disastrous consequences. It was a striking example of a dramatised 'what if?' scenario, but the fictional programme immediately became the subject of a serious *Newsnight* discussion, where experts pontificated on whether its fantastic scenario was 'plausible' or not.

Since then, the BBC has launched an entire genre of Apocalypse-light entertainment shows, screening docudramas about a smallpox epidemic in Britain and a dirty-bomb attack on London, along with a series about similarly speculative risks entitled *If....* These programmes projected some of society's current fears into the near future, and asked what would happen if the worst possibility became reality. So we were treated to dramatised considerations of what would happen *if* the lights went out, *if* we don't stop eating and so on. These were presented not as horror-film-style fantasies, but as real risks – an impression reinforced by the involvement of genuine experts in the shows. The professor of food policy who says of obesity, 'This slaughter cannot go on!' in 'If... We Don't Stop Eating' is the same man who in real life dreamed up the far fetched proposal for a fatty-food tax that was almost taken up by the government. The series editor on *If...* insisted that the filmmakers were no more guilty of scaremongering than government emergency planners, British Telecom or the CIA when they create speculative 'what if?' scenarios. He was right about that, at least.

Almost every day, it seems, we are confronted with fresh evidence of how far the obsession with risk and risk-aversion has gone. It all goes to reinforce my view that this has now become the major barrier to social, scientific and technological advance. It is humanity's most powerful self-imposed constraint on its own potential liberation. A century or more ago, an atheistic humanist such as myself might have said that organised religion played that role. Half a century or more ago, it might have been right-wing nationalism or Stalinism, depending on the circumstances. Now I see it as risk aversion, the culture of fear and the politics of organised paranoia.

As the old political and religious systems have lost their purchase on society in recent times, risk and precaution have emerged as the focus for an attempt to create a new kind of morality to guide human behaviour. Safety-first has become a virtue for its own sake, to be repeated like a religious mantra, regardless of the practical consequences. And, especially since 9/11 brought these underlying trends to the surface of society, organised paranoia has now become a policy principle guiding government planning and discussion.

In the run-up to the 2003 Panic Attack conference, *spiked* asked leading scientists to name any historic advances that they thought could not have been made if the 'precautionary principle' which constrains science and technology today had been in place in the past. They came up with a scary list, starting with A for aspirin and going through to X for X-rays.

Yet the better-safe-than-sorry spirit of the precautionary principle is not confined to the scientific sphere. It has escaped from the laboratory to infect public discussion about everything from how we should raise our children to how armies ought to fight wars. When the quasi-religious belief in safety-first touches so many disparate issues, from mobile-phone masts to GM foods, it is clear that the problem must be bigger than the science of the specific disputes. It is feeding off far wider cultural assumptions about human vulnerability, and our supposed incapacity to cope with risk and uncertainty. This is what is really new.

Humanity has always faced risks, and there has always been a debate about how to manage them. Today, however, unlike in the past, risk is seen not as something we can handle or perhaps even turn into opportunity, but as something that we suffer from and must be guarded against.

The war on terror has become the latest focus for much of this stuff. Take the memorable statement made by one British security official, after the alleged discovery of the chemical agent ricin in a London flat, that 'There is a very serious threat out there still that chemicals that have not yet been found may be used by people who have not yet been identified' (*Financial Times*, 8 January 2003). As terrorism expert Bill Durodie commented, this is now 'the logic of our times: never mind the evidence, just focus on the possibility'.

George W Bush and Tony Blair have been accused of exploiting the politics of fear around the war on terror. Yet many critics of the US and UK governments seem perfectly willing to deploy the politics of fear in their own arguments. Thus, David Corn, editor of *The Nation*, America's leading left-leaning journal, argues that 'technologies long challenged by environmental advocates are potential sources of immense danger in an era of terrorism'. Americans for Fuel-Efficient Cars also link their campaign against sports utility vehicles (SUVs) to people's fear of terrorism, arguing that Americans should 'free ourselves from the nations and terrorists holding us hostage through our addiction to oil'.

Who really benefits from this increasingly pervasive culture of fear, the belief in human vulnerability and the politics of organised paranoia? Apart perhaps from some compensation lawyers or paper-mask manufacturers, nobody does really. The elevation of safety-first into an absolute virtue disorientates society to the point where a one-off accident can close down an entire railway system, or where senior judges can refuse to consider parole for a man who shot a burglar on the grounds that he may pose a risk to others who try to burgle his home.

Even the New Labour government can discover that the precautionary principle comes back to bite it from behind. When the global SARS panic broke, the British authorities tried to reassure the public that there was no real risk in this country. But, having already put Britain on a permanent state of alert about the alleged threat of bioterrorism, they could not get away with such a sensibly low-key response. Immediately, the government found itself accused of complacency and of putting the public at risk by not doing enough in the way of airport checks and quarantine. On this, as on many other risk-related issues, the Tory opposition proved that there are now no depths to which it will not sink in search of a populist cause. Organised paranoia has caused New Labour even more trouble with regard to the MMR triple vaccination, as the government's promotion of innumerable other health panics over everything from passive smoking to fast food made many people less willing to accept official assurances that MMR is safe.

The fact that people in our society now live longer, healthier lives and enjoy a better diet than ever before would surely be seen as a cause for celebration in a more level-headed present. Instead, we seem obsessed with worrying about these things, through panics about the supposed 'demographic time bomb' or 'obesity time bomb'. According to the doctrine of organised paranoia, everything now has to be for the worst, in the worst of all possible worlds.

Writing about the panic over AIDS in the late 1980s, the recently deceased American critic Susan Sontag noted how a widespread 'sense of cultural distress or failure' was encouraging continual 'fantasies of doom'. In this peculiarly modern mood of social pessimism, the end is believed to be nigh but never comes. It is a case, as she put it, not so much of 'Apocalypse Now', but of 'Apocalypse From Now On'. Sontag saw the consequence of living in this perpetual state of fear as 'an unparalleled violence that is being done to our sense of reality, our humanity'.

Challenging organised paranoia and all the rest of this risk-averse irrationalism should be a priority for anybody concerned about social and scientific advance. To do nothing in the face of this danger would be to risk squandering the great potential for society to change and move forward, and that is one risk that it is really not worth running. The cultural mood that Sontag described so well poses a more pressing threat to civilised life as we know it than could any speculative 'what if?' scenario.

PART ONE:

HOW PEOPLE
GET IT WRONG

Chapter One

WHOSE OPINION CAN WE TRUST?

BY STANLEY FELDMAN AND VINCENT MARKS

Frederick II of Germany wrote in the thirteenth century: 'One ought not to believe anything, save that which can be proven by nature and the force of reason.' His views were echoed in the sixteenth century by the French essayist Michel de Montaigne: 'I would have every man write of that which he knows.' The implication was that one must distinguish between opinion, which is that which one thinks may be true, and fact. Only opinion based on fact is a truly worthy basis for promulgating new ideas. Using observed fact to test opinion was the basis of the essay format. The word itself comes from the French verb *essayer*, to test or try, and it was the essay form that Montaigne used as a means of trying out his own ideas.

Today, it is all too common to find would-be Montaignes using opinion as though it were fact as a basis for their essays. This leaves us with the difficult problem of separating fact from opinion. If two people present diverging views on a subject, who should one trust? Which one is presenting fact and which opinion?

This should be a relatively simple exercise but, because of sophistry, spin and the deliberate misinterpretation of information, it has become increasing difficult to distinguish true facts from the plethora of dubious opinions with which we are bombarded. Fact is verifiable information, numbers or results that can be reproduced. Unfortunately, the misinformation explosion has swamped factual stories. The improbable sells more newspapers than the probable, and the more times an improbable, unsupported story is reported, the more it enters into the folklore of 'everybody knows that...' Ask anyone how many people died in the Chernobyl disaster and the response is likely to be that 'everyone knows' it was hundreds or thousands. We have been deliberately led into believing this story by those opposed to nuclear energy. In fact, the World Health Organisation reported in 2003 that there were fewer than 40 deaths in the 20 years following the disaster. Although there was a significant increase in the number of cases of cancer of the thyroid, there was not any increase noticed in the incidence of leukaemia.

Who is going to give us accurate, unbiased information that we can trust? We should be able to trust the various British government bodies and the BBC. Unfortunately, even these usually reliable sources fall into the misinformation trap. The BBC, the government, the chief medical officer and the Food Standards Agency, to take some examples, do not set out to be partisan or to push deliberate falsehoods, but the information presented by these authoritative bodies is subject to the bias of the presenter and his or her particular interpretation of information. The result is that opinion becomes presented as fact.

There seems to be a mistaken belief within the BBC that equal weight must be given to both sides of a problem. The author Douglas Adams put it succinctly when he wrote in *The Salmon of Doubt*, 'All opinions are not equal. Some are a great deal more robust, sophisticated and well supported in logic and argument than others.' The concept that fair play demands that all opinions be treated equally is nonsense. But today we frequently see warriors against reason paraded as heroes on the BBC, representing this or that irrational pressure group. The BBC gives them credibility. *You and Yours* recently gave air time to an advocate of coffee enemas for the treatment of cancer, who failed to adequately explain why taking coffee by this somewhat curious route should be better than taking it by mouth. By giving this contributor the same opportunity as an expert to present a totally ludicrous opinion on the air, the BBC implied that his views have the same legitimacy as those of an informed spokesman on the subject. The BBC bestows an undeserved and inappropriate authority on the warriors against reason. Their ideas gain an undeserved credence as a result of the media obsession with providing a 'balanced debate'.

Even government reports are subject to opinion presented as fact. The government warning against added salt sits uneasily with its advice to replace both the water and salt lost in hot weather, and also with the statement in its own briefing document, published by the Parliamentary Office of Science and Technology in 2004, that the 'Intersalt study (1997), the largest ever carried out, found no correlation between salt intake and blood pressure'. The report of a government select committee in 2004, as reported by the BBC, stated that obesity has increased 400 per cent in 25 years – when the present standard measurement of obesity, the Body Mass Index (BMI), has only been used for about 17 years. Before that time, it was the Metropolitan Life Insurance Company tables that were used (see *Obesity* p.53).

This, then, is the problem: how do we know that what we are being told is reliable and factual? The first step is to exclude the phonies – the flat-earth society proponents and those who claim that meditation, wearing blue beads or standing on your head for half an hour each day will cure cancer. Their ideas are so ludicrous that they can be readily spotted. It is a failing of our society, with all its laws to protect the consumer, that we allow such charlatans to prey upon the desperate plight of sick or ignorant people.

More plausible are the self-promoting experts who try to scare us by stories of impending doom. They talk in meaningless slogans like 'freeing your spiritual self' (from what, one asks?), 'concreting over the countryside' (looking down on the British countryside from an aeroplane at a few hundred feet, it looks as verdant as anywhere on earth), 'Frankenstein foods' (GM food has been on sale in many countries for eight years and no ill effect has been reported), 'epidemic of obesity' (but one that has been going on for 40 years) and so on. The ideas behind their slogans are scientifically improbable, but refuting them with absolute certainty is virtually impossible. So, when an interviewer asks a scientist, 'Can you rule out the possibility that London may be flooded in the future?', to which the scientist of course cannot categorically answer 'No', this results in the headline: 'SCIENTIST CONFIRMS LONDON MAY FLOOD'.

Having eliminated the peddlers of the irrational, one is left with the advocates of the plausible. Unless one is particularly well informed, one has to rely on the advice of an expert as to what is likely to be fact and what is opinion. The problem, then, is who is an expert? By and large the older, major universities are more demanding in the qualifications of their academic staff than the smaller, newer ones, and the older mainstream areas of study have a more predictable level of scientific attainment. The expert from an established university is likely to be more reliable, although he or she may be more reluctant to accept valid but novel or iconoclastic ideas. Few of us can check the curriculum vitae of or the source of information used by the expert, but in certain circumstances credibility can be inferred from the publication in which it appeared. *Figure 1* indicates a progression of reliability from information in peer-reviewed journals to statements by propagandists and pressure groups.

Medicine is a more rigorous course of study than that of nursing or one of the allied therapies. It is reasonable, therefore, to believe that the opinion of a doctor is more likely to be credible than that of a therapist. Like all broad generalisations, this is subject to notable exceptions, but there is no essential course of study that qualifies one to be called a 'health expert', or to call oneself a 'non-interventionist surgeon'. It is not necessary to study human physiology to become an expert on nutrition or food (indeed the chairman of the Food Standards Agency who is an expert, is a zoologist), whereas one has

FIGURE 1

Type of information	Type of author	Type of publication	Intended audience
Primary	Scientists and epidemiologists	Research papers in peer-reviewed journals	Other researchers in the same field
Secondary	Research and academic scientists	Scientific reviews in peer-reviewed journals	Academics and teachers
Tertiary	Academic authors and scientists; expert committees	Monographs, textbooks, consensus reports	Students, practitioners and popularists
Quaternary	Popularists	Books for the layman, science-based radio and TV programmes and interviews	'Intellectual' members of the public
Quinternary	Journalists	Newspapers, TV and radio, magazines,	The public
Sexternary	Copywriters	Adverts and editorials	Intended customers
Septernary	Propagandists	Press statements, interviews	The public
Others: folklore, shop assistants, 'health writers'			

to follow an essential core course of scientific study in order to become a doctor. Academic doctors are not necessarily more expert than practising ones, but because of the nature of their work they are more likely to question an opinion and to be more demanding in the standard of evidence before they will accept a statement as true.

Life would be much simpler and safer if we could immediately recognise an expert and rely upon their views as being authoritative. This was the concept behind the Lord Chief Justice's plea for arbitration panels to appoint a single expert witness whose opinion would be accepted by all. This would work if all expert opinions were based on agreed fact. Unfortunately, when it comes to interpreting the meaning of the facts, it becomes a matter of individual, fallible opinion. As a result, this worthy notion has had a limited impact, and we still have gladiatorial contests in all criminal cases and some civil ones between the opposing opinions of experts, a battle for the most believable or the most glib.

So, how can we assess the views with which we are bombarded? We have to start by separating fact from opinion, then assess the reasonableness of interpretation of the evidence against scientific probability. Fact is something that is proven and can be reproduced; opinion relies on a belief by the person making the proposition rather than proof of the proposal. We should ignore presentational gimmicks and slogans, and look for the core message. We have to assess the credibility and bias of the messenger along with his message.

In the preparation of this book, we have asked the authors to present what is known or is generally accepted as factual and to separate it from what they consider probable. Scientists are aware that many of the commonly accepted beliefs in healthcare are based on misapprehensions which need to be exposed to scientific scrutiny. For this purpose, we have asked our panel of scientists, whom we consider to be expert, to write 'that which they know'.

At the end of the day, we must remember that, in the world of healthcare, things are getting better. The fact that we are living longer, healthier lives suggests that there cannot be anything terribly wrong with the air we breathe, the food we eat or the way we live.

We must remember this in spite of the blandishments, threats, warnings and various campaigns by governments to make us eat this diet or that, to forgo a familiar habit or to exercise ourselves until we drop. It is a sobering thought, first expressed by John Locke in 1689 in his treatise 'A Letter Concerning Toleration': 'No man can be forced to be healthful, whether he will or no.' In a free society, individuals must judge for themselves what information they choose to heed, and what they ignore.

Chapter Two

THE MISUSE OF NUMBERS

BY STANLEY FELDMAN AND VINCENT MARKS

'There are three kinds of lies: lies,
damned lies, and statistics.'

MARK TWAIN

'THIRTY THOUSAND PEOPLE DIE EACH YEAR FROM EATING TOO MUCH FAT', splashed the headlines in a recent newspaper article – but what would happen if they *stopped* eating too much fat? Would they live forever, or would they succumb to something else within the same time frame? The answer is of course that they would die of something else, possibly even sooner than if they kept on eating fat. How did anyone come up with this number anyway? Has anyone – let alone 30,000 people – ever had their cause of death certified as being due to eating too much fat? The truth is that this figure, like so many, is pure speculation.

The media should carry a health warning: 'Statistics can damage your life'. Pressure groups, spin doctors and even Members of Parliament use figures in such a loose way that numbers, which have an exact meaning, become vague, imprecise or deliberately misleading. Take, for example, the headline that 'UP TO 60% OF THE

POPULATION DOES NOT UNDERSTAND THE PROPOSED EU CONSTITUTION'.
The statement conveys the impression that the EU constitution
baffles most people. This may be right – but it could also mean that
as few as 5 per cent or as many as 60 per cent are confused by it.
When this careless use of numbers is applied to medical and social
problems, the result can cause unnecessary alarm, silly therapeutic
interventions or a large expenditure on an insignificant problem. Let
us examine some examples of the misleading use of numbers.

'UP TO'

The animal-welfare pressure group WWF-UK suggested in June 2004
that global warming would wipe out 'up to one million species of
wildlife by 2050'. This conclusion is based on a worst-case scenario
occurring at every turn. It can only be arrived at by taking the highest
figure for global warming, which is 10 times greater than the more
realistic ones, an inability of any species to adapt and the loss of a
favourable habitat for all species occurring at the same time, whereas
it is likely that what is bad for one species may be good for another.
The only purpose of this absurd statistic is to frighten the unwary.
The author of the original report, himself an environmental
campaigner, complained that the press release was 'a woeful
misrepresentation of science' by the pressure group. He had actually
suggested in his report that as few as 5 per cent or as many as 78 per
cent of this number of species could be at risk.

BASELINE BIAS

Baseline bias is another way of bamboozling the public and is
commonly used by the financial-service industry to convey a
misleading impression. Let us say the cost of a barrel of oil has
increased from $10 to $45 since 1945. If you want to sell a gas-
guzzling aeroplane, you could start a price comparison in 1973, at
the time of the Suez crisis, and close it just before the present surge
in oil prices. You could then draw a graph showing that, in the 30-
year period covered, the price of oil increased by less than inflation.

Baseline bias is a favourite trick of environmental pressure groups. By taking a starting point some 250 years ago, you can demonstrate a highly worrying increase in average world temperature. It becomes much less alarming if you start 50 or 100 years ago, and minimal if you start in Roman times when there were vineyards as far north as York. The reason is that 250 years ago just happened to see some of the coldest winters of the millennium. The summer of 2003 was particular warm – certainly warmer than 2002 and 2004. What if 2005 is even colder than 2004? Does this mean that we will have to abandon all our theories of global warming, just as we did the forecasts of an impending ice age made just 30 or 40 years ago, based on a run of unusually cold years. How long do we wait until we decide the planet is merely emerging, somewhat erratically, from the last ice age and not really getting much warmer? The secret lies in the starting point, or baseline: something as slow to change as global temperature has to be measured in thousands, not just hundreds, of years if it is to show any meaningful trends. The great debate about CO_2 and global warming is a distraction from the real problem of our reliance on fossil fuels and what will happen when we have used them all up.

Similarly, the decline in atmospheric pollution in London over the past three years is not very impressive, but if one goes back 50 years it is dramatic. The reason for this is that we have succeeded in reducing the major pollutants to such a low level that the rate of improvement has inevitably tailed off, as it always does. Improvements always follow the law of diminishing returns which says that as you near perfection the benefit you obtain from an increased effort becomes smaller and smaller. Perfection is never attainable, however nice it might be to think that it is.

EXTRAPOLATION

Unless you are aware that figures quoted in an article are an extrapolation beyond the data available, you can be fooled into believing that a catastrophe is just around the corner.

Remember when the number of patients with new variant Creutzfeldt-Jakob disease was going to reach 100,000 or so within a few years of its discovery? In fact, the total number of patients dying from all types of Creutzfeldt-Jakob disease has more or less reached a plateau and is very few more than before the BSE crisis began. A recent revival of the scare predicted that 10,000 UK citizens might die from BSE. It appears to have been based on extrapolating from a sample of about 2,000 tonsils that were examined for the BSE prion (a protein particle which is believed to cause the disease). The study revealed one positive and two suspicious tonsils which, if true for the whole of the population of the UK, provides the figure of 10,000 potentially infected people. Extrapolation is always chancy, but when it is based on such a small number of cases it is not only meaningless, but also potentially dangerous.

A recent article in a newspaper said that 40,000 patients might be dying each year from the side-effects of drugs in hospitals (*The Times*, August 2004). The figure was derived by extrapolating from a single hospital study of the deaths of 28 patients in whom a side-effect of a drug, however unimportant, was recorded at some time during their treatment and who eventually died in the hospital. Included in the deaths were patients who would have died of the disease for which the drugs were being prescribed in any case. No allowance was made for the proportion of the particular hospital's population that was made up of those who were especially vulnerable, such as the very old and sick. One can immediately see the danger of extrapolating from the results of one small study to the whole country. Patients do undoubtedly die from the side-effects of drugs. These are, however, carefully monitored and responsibly reported and do not yield the scary figures quoted in *The Times*.

In recent times, in order to meet this criticism, it has become common to find several separate small studies joined together and presented as a large-scale investigation. This is termed meta-analysis. Unless all these studies have been conducted on similar populations using the same methods, however, their results are seldom more reliable than that of the weakest study among them.

The advent of computers, with their ability to perform in a few minutes complex mathematical calculations that would previously have taken hours, days or even years, has encouraged a form of mathematical extrapolation called modelling. Modelling can magnify any lack of precision in the subject modelled and amplify the effect of any mistaken assumptions. It is responsible for many of the exaggerated predictions about trends that that are likely to occur in the future, sometimes on the flimsiest of data. It has been described as a pop-art form since it takes an actual situation and tries to reproduce it artificially on a much larger scale.

COMPARING LIKE WITH LIKE

An environmental pressure group recently claimed that atmospheric pollution in London kills the equivalent number of people each year as would die if two jumbo jets crashed. This scare story originated in a report from the Department of Health which found that in the very hot summer of 2003 there were 800 more deaths than were expected. The pressure group suggested that these deaths were due to ozone pollution.

However, the people who would die in an aeroplane crash are, by and large, young and active and would have expected another 20 to 40 years of life, while those who died during the heatwave were elderly, terminally sick patients with breathing problems who had a life expectancy measured in months. In comparing the numbers who died, in these two situations, the environmentalists were deliberately comparing the wrong things: they should not have been comparing the numbers of deaths but the loss of years of expected life. They were comparing apples with oranges. Of course, there are also other possible causes of death during a heatwave. Most of the deaths that occurred in the elderly in Paris during the hot summer of 2003, where the death toll was much higher than in London, were found to have been due to dehydration.

THE SIGNIFICANCE OF 'SIGNIFICANCE'

The word 'significant' means different things to statisticians and laymen. To the layman something is significant if it is big and important. To the statistician and scientist the deviation between two observations is significant only if it reflects a genuine difference between those measurements, rather than one that is down to chance or an error of measurement. Most science involves making measurements, but measurements are never quite as precise or exact as we would like them to be. Two numbers may differ from one another either because of the difficulty of making the measurement or because there is a real difference between them. It may be comparatively simple to measure the length of a piece of string and compare it with the length of another piece of string, but how do you measure the rainfall in one year and compare it with another, or measure whether a new drug is statistically better for treating an illness than one that was formerly available?

Take multiple sclerosis, for example. This slowly progressive illness can last 40 years or more, and be punctuated by remarkable spontaneous remissions during which the patient may return, without any outside intervention, to a state indistinguishable from 'normal'. How, in these circumstances, can you be sure that your new treatment works? In order to find out, it is necessary to conduct a randomised, controlled clinical trial in which the benefits of the new treatment are compared with those produced by a placebo, or with the best available treatment, given under exactly the same conditions. But what will you use to judge the success of the drug? Clearly you cannot rely on just how the patient feels, because improvement might be due to a spontaneous remission. Suppose that a remission occurred within one month of starting treatment in 60 out of the 100 patients given the new drug, but only in 55 of those given the alternative treatment: how can you be sure that the additional benefit was due to the drug and did not reflect a chance occurrence or an unintentional difference between the patients in each group?

Using appropriate mathematical formulae, the probability of the difference being pure chance can be calculated. If it is less than 1 in 20 the difference is said, by convention, to be 'significant'. If the probability is less than 1 in 100, it would be described as 'very significant', and so on – the terminology becoming stronger as the probability of the difference being due to chance becomes smaller. All that 'significant' means is that the drug did have an effect, even if it was not a very profound one, and it certainly does not mean that it had an effect on everyone. It might also happen that after a year the group receiving the supposedly active treatment was no better off than those receiving the placebo. They may, in fact, be worse off. Yet such a treatment would undoubtedly be described in the newspapers as 'a major breakthrough'.

WHAT IS NORMAL?

What happens when we want to define 'normal'? To most of us, normal means typical and healthy. To the statistician, it means

FIGURE 2

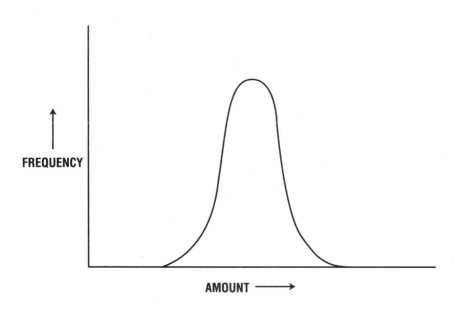

A normal distribution curve.

something else. It describes a distribution of measurements which, when plotted on graph paper, gives rise to a typical bell-shaped curve (*Figure 2*). By convention, everything in the tails of the curves – the lowest 2.5 per cent and the highest 2.5 per cent – is called 'abnormal'. Using this criterion, someone who is 6 foot 6 inches tall is 'abnormally tall', but it is of no clinical consequence. Just being abnormal does not mean that you are ill or about to become so.

A recent newspaper story suggested that carrying a mobile phone might cause sterility. It was based on the tentative findings of a small study in Europe which found a decrease of up to 30 per cent in the sperm count of people carrying a mobile phone compared with a control group who did not. The difference was statistically highly significant. However, while carrying a mobile phone might possibly be clinically relevant to men on the borderline of fertility who are in their prime reproductive years, it would be of no relevance to most men who produce a massive superfluity of sperm. After all, it only needs one sperm to fertilise an ovum.

This brings us to consider who the 'average man' we hear so much about actually is. People and things may be 'typical' or 'representative', but surely never average. This is a mathematical term and applies only to numbers. Take the newspaper headline 'FIFTY PER CENT OF DOCTORS PERFORM LESS WELL THAN AVERAGE'. It gives the reader the impression that all is not well with the practice of medicine. In fact, it only states the obvious, since 50 per cent must, by definition, perform better than the mean average and so 50 per cent will perform less well – but only if you can find a way of expressing performance numerically.

Comparing averages can be very misleading. If little Johnny scored 60 per cent in his exams when the class average was 50 per cent, it might sound as if his performance was quite satisfactory. But if, say, three out of the 11 boys in the class scored less than 5 per cent, it would have a huge effect on the average mark and Johnny may have scored less well than almost everybody else in the class.

A more useful statistic, then, would be to compare the scores achieved by an equal number of students.

When we are told that 60 per cent of children are overweight, this statistic compares each child to an 'ideal' weight rather than to an 'average' weight. It is a seemingly shocking statistic, and one which might lead us to believe that the 'epidemic of obesity' we always hear about is genuinely upon us. In fact, the statistic tells us almost nothing. Leaving aside the fact that this ideal weight is entirely subjective, it is self-evident that those who are only a few ounces, or even a few pounds, over the 'ideal' weight run a relatively small risk of any adverse effects on their health; it is those who are much heavier who are at risk of their lives being shortened by obesity. But the statistic gives us no idea of how many children are slightly overweight and how many are seriously overweight. What it does do, on the other hand, is serve to scare us and to sell newspapers.

CIRCUMSTANTIAL EVIDENCE

Many of the scare stories that appear in the media start with an epidemiological study. These compare the rate, occurrence or coincidence of two events. Some of these studies are very good, with great care being taken to prevent bias and to limit the effect of outside factors. Nevertheless, they all end up trying to demonstrate an association between a potentially causative factor and an effect. The problem with these sorts of studies, however, is that by itself the association between the events is circumstantial and says nothing about their causal relationship to one another. Take the example given by Darrell Huff in his book *How to Lie with Statistics*: the greatest number of suicides in the UK occur in June; June is also the most popular month for marriages. Does this mean that these two events are related?

BIAS

Many studies depend upon the reports of individuals. The results of such studies are often subject to bias, particularly when they are based on telephone or postal questionnaires. If a study trying to find out if a particular detergent caused skin irritation was carried out by post, it is likely that someone not troubled by skin irritation would throw the letter in the bin, whereas someone *with* skin irritation would reply. Unless there was a very high return rate, the results would be subject to bias and be meaningless.

A recent postal questionnaire sent out by the Home Office reported that 1 in 20 women had been raped. This result is intuitively unlikely, and the nature of the questionnaire was bound to give the result it did. The chances of happily married women who have never been raped replying to the questionnaire were very small. In addition, if the definition of rape was not well defined, it is not beyond the bounds of possibility that some women, perhaps those in an unhappy relationship, will have answered the question '*Do you believe you have been raped?*' rather than '*Have you been raped?*' which is very different. The disturbing aspect of this study was not just the waste of taxpayers' money, but the fact that the results are likely to be used as the basis for legislation.

Telephone studies are just as likely to be subject to bias, as the respondent invariably tries to give the questioner the answer that they think he or she wants to hear.

UNBALANCING THE EQUATION

Benjamin, age five, casually remarked, 'God eats a lot of fish.' The background to this improbable assertion was his mother's remark that fish is good for your brain. His tendentious reasoning was that 'God must be very clever because he can hear what we are saying no matter what language we use', it follows therefore that 'he must eat a lot of fish'. A byline in the *Sunday Times* (August 2004) indicated that salt causes intellectual failure. It appears an investigation in Boston showed, in a trial of 2,500 people, that high blood pressure was correlated with minor strokes, and minor strokes could cause intellectual degeneration, which is not unreasonable. The author, having believing that salt can cause high blood pressure wrote up the story to implicate salt as the cause of intellectual degeneration. This piece of tendentious reporting ignores the evidence that the Japanese, who eat twice as much salt as an American on average, are no less clever and live longer lives.

Then there are numbers apparently picked out of the air but repeated so many times that they develop an authority of their own. A letter from Transport for London says that 20,000 people die each year from atmospheric pollution in London. In fact, pollution in London is now lower than it has been for centuries. It is possible that a few with severe respiratory diseases are made worse by diesel fumes from lorries and buses but these are patients on the edge of breathing failure who would not be made better even if they lived in a plastic bubble fed with filtered air. These figures are frankly false but because they go unchallenged become accepted as fact.

With all the numbers that are bandied about to show this disease or that food is killing us we should remember that we are living longer, healthier lives and that 'life itself is a fatal disease' if we do not die of one thing it will increase the death rate from an alternative.

Chapter Three

EPIDEMIOLOGY

BY STANLEY FELDMAN

In the criminal court it is necessary that the case against the plaintiff should be proved 'beyond reasonable doubt' before anyone is found guilty. Even in the civil court, where the onus of proof is reduced, it is necessary to convince the jury that the case has been established 'on the balance of probabilities'. Even these rigorous requirements have not stopped occasional prosecutions from succeeding, only for it to be shown at a later date that the level of proof was inadequate or flawed.

When it comes to medicine and healthcare however, circumstantial evidence, sometimes of the most tendentious nature, is frequently accepted as sufficient proof for health campaigns that may affect the lifestyle of many, leading to the appointment of 'health tsars' to oversee these changes and the vilification of anyone who opposes them. The research that generates this circumstantial evidence is called 'epidemiology'.

Epidemiology sets out to show a meaningful correlation between a particular circumstance and an event that subsequently occurs. If a positive association is uncovered, it is implied that the circumstance studied is the cause of that event. By itself, such an association can only be circumstantial and should never be accepted as sufficient proof of a relationship between the cause and the effect.

Not all epidemiological research comes up with the wrong answers – it often points the researcher in the right direction. But, by itself, it cannot prove anything beyond reasonable doubt. It has produced notable successes suggesting that there is a correlation between a particular disease state and a causative factor, but even the best of these studies only produces evidence that is circumstantial and needs to be subjected to further investigation in order to prove a point. No epidemiological study should be accepted as proof, or its results propagated, until supportive evidence is available. This is particularly true when the results run counter to intuitive reason.

Many years ago, in the mid-nineteenth century, Professor Robert Koch, the discoverer of the bacillus that causes tuberculosis, enumerated the necessary conditions for proof that condition A was caused by B. The most important of these was that:

The causative factor B must always be present in condition A.
Removing the causative factor B must lessen or cure condition A.
Reintroducing B must reproduce A.

Merely demonstrating a statistical relationship between A and B comes nowhere near the standard that Koch required for proof, no matter how carefully the conditions are controlled or what allowance is made in the study to offset any potential source of bias. A casual coincidence between two events remains circumstantial until a causative relationship is proved or Koch's three principal conditions of proof are fulfilled.

EPIDEMIOLOGICAL SUCCESSES

In 1854, John Snow removed the handle of the water pump in Broad Street, London. This was the first significant adventure in epidemiology and earned him the sobriquet of 'the father of epidemiology'. Snow had observed that, in his Soho Parish, those who drew their water from the Broad Street pump suffered a very high incidence of cholera, while neighbours who used another nearby pump, with water coming from another source, did not. He removed the pump handle to stop people using water from the suspect pump. The incidence of new cases of cholera fell to one, and that case had used old contaminated water. This provided Snow with proof that the source of the cholera was in the water coming from the pump. His idea was not predicated on the removal of the pump handle, nor was it proof of the cause of cholera. His study had shown that cholera occurred in those drinking water from the Broad Street pump, and that removing this source stopped the disease. He had demonstrated two of Koch's postulates. Epidemiological research of this sort, used to support or disprove a theory, is valuable and its results constitute legitimate proof.

In 1956, Richard Doll and Austin Bradford Hill published their epoch-making epidemiological study on smoking and cancer of the lung. This alerted us to the very real dangers of smoking. By comparing two very large groups of reasonably matched adults, Doll was able to demonstrate a dramatically increased risk of cancer of the lungs in smokers. What gave this study credence, raising it above the level of circumstantial evidence, was that he showed that the risk increased with the number of cigarettes smoked and the duration of smoking. It was dose related. His results fitted in with scientific and intuitive reasoning. However, it remained only a casual association until it was demonstrated that those who stopped smoking dramatically reduced the risk of developing cancer of the lung. This later study fulfilled Koch's second postulate. No doubt if it had been ethical to reintroduce smoking in those who had given it up, the third postulate could also have been demonstrated.

TOO MANY VARIABLES

If we compare these studies with more recent ones that have been used to justify attempts to coerce behavioural changes or social changes, we begin to see the limitations of epidemiological evidence.

Several epidemiological studies have demonstrated an association between income and longevity of life. It has been deduced from these that poverty causes disease. This conclusion is intuitively suspect, as the actual causes of many of the common diseases are known and only casually related to the income of those who suffer them. The definition of poverty keeps changing: it varies from place to place and is not necessarily a reflection of income but rather of a way of life. There are many different causes of poverty, and its effects are far from uniform. Poverty may be caused by the disease itself, which may limit the patient's ability to work. A low income in one group may be associated with insanitary housing, while in another it may be reflected in the diet. It is impossible to separate any one cause or to produce evidence of any particular element, such as bad housing, poor level of knowledge, unhealthy lifestyle, depression, bad diet or an ethnic genetic susceptibility, because of the lack of specificity in the study. As a result these studies are impossible to interpret in a scientifically meaningful manner. There is little evidence that removing these people from poverty reverses the reduced life expectancy, at least in the short term. The association between poverty and health shown in these studies is undoubtedly valid, but it cannot be taken as proven evidence that it is the poverty itself, the low income, that is the cause of a shortened life expectancy.

If one takes a blunderbuss approach to a disease and casts one's net too wide by studying all the possible circumstances with which it could be associated, one of them is likely to show a positive correlation with something – but this does not constitute evidence that it alone is the cause of the problem. One such study, after discarding all the factors that failed to demonstrate a positive correlation, found an association between pesticide in food and brain tumours. The view was then promulgated that pesticides caused tumours of the brain. However, it ignored the absence of an increased incidence of brain tumours in crop-sprayers, the group of people exposed to the greatest dose of pesticides for the longest period.

Those advocating a ban on smoking in public places quote an

epidemiological study reported in 2004 indicating a link between parental smoking habits and childhood asthma. Smoking, for all its ill effects on health, has never been implicated as a cause of asthma; indeed, before 1960, when cigarette smoking was widespread, the incidence of childhood asthma was much lower than at present. Another study found that passive smoking was more dangerous than actually inhaling the smoke directly. The laws of physics dictate that the concentration of any noxious substance contained in the smoke would decrease by the square of the distance it travelled. It would be four times less when the distance was doubled, and 16 times more dilute when the range was increased fourfold. Common sense suggests that the conclusions drawn from these studies are wrong. While one can sympathise with the objectives of those trying to dissuade people from smoking, this should not involve bad science.

META-ANALYSIS

This important-sounding technique hides a statistical trick that is commonly used to support tendentious epidemiological results. It combines the results of several studies so as to boost the numbers, the so-called 'power' of the investigation. It is a technique that is open to abuse. By combining the results of 10 bad studies, it is suggested, we end up with one good one. The methods used in the various studies often differ significantly, as do the methods used for the collection of data, the criteria for inclusion in the investigation and the numbers involved. The end result is then rehashed as additional new evidence, which can now be said to be 'supported by the work of many scientists'. It is frequently used to lump studies together so as to disguise their individual weaknesses.

BAD SCIENCE

Another example of the failure to encompass the complexity of the problem being studied and, as a result, coming to the wrong conclusion occurred in 1954 in the USA. Two eminent doctors from the Massachusetts General Hospital, Beecher and Todd, investigated the effect of the introduction of curare, a muscle-relaxant drug, on anaesthetic mortality. Their large study was carried out in 10 US teaching institutions. Beecher and Todd found that the mortality rate associated with the use of curare was four times higher in the patients receiving the drug than in the control patients who did not receive curare. As a result, they concluded that the use of curare was lethal. The use of curare fell dramatically and it was many years before its use was re-established in America.

The results ran counter to the experience in the UK, where curare was used in far bigger doses than in America and in a greater variety of cases. Beecher and Todd came to a suspect conclusion – they seemed to have ignored the effect on anaesthetic mortality of the *way* the drug was being used. The students and nurses who used the drug most frequently in America were not sufficiently trained, and they did not appreciate the need for artificial ventilation or the need to reverse any residual effect of the drug at the end of an operation. It was not the drug that killed patients; it was the way it was used.

UNLIKELY RESULTS

Too small a study, or a freak sample group, can reveal coincidences that defy reason. The extrapolation of the results obtained from a specific study to a wider, general population can produce unjustified conclusions.

If I were to carry out a study of the number of gooseberry bushes in Richmond and the number of babies born, and came up with a positive correlation between the two, few people would start believing that babies were found under gooseberry bushes. Yet people seem ready to believe the improbable when some epidemiological questionnaire carried out for someone's PhD thesis comes up with equivalent nonsense. A similar study on the effect of atmospheric pollution on childhood asthma might reveal that, as pollution levels fell, the incidence of asthma increased. A further analysis would show that in the last few years, the rate of improvement in the quality of the atmosphere has decreased and the number of new cases of asthma has also declined. This epidemiological study would be forced to conclude that atmospheric pollution prevented childhood asthma. This is clearly unlikely. It is often the very improbability of the result that gives it publicity, and it is the publicity that gives it credibility. A recent study apparently suggested that the use of antiperspirants could cause cancer of the breast. This is intuitive nonsense. Even if antiperspirants did influence the incidence of the disease, it would require an enormous study over 20 years to determine any contributory effect. Similarly, the extrapolation of the results of a well-designed study on long-term hormone-replacement therapy (HRT), with a combination of drugs hardly ever used today, to the risk associated with current medication caused a panic in all users of HRT.

Just as misleading is the generalisation made from studies of an effect in an artificially restricted area, or with a particular causative factor. One of the most influential of these studies was the demonstration of clusters of children with leukaemia in certain areas near the Sellafield nuclear reprocessing plant. This has been extrapolated to suggest that nuclear anything causes leukaemia. It has fuelled the totally irrational fear of nuclear energy. There is plenty of good scientific evidence that there is no correlation between a low background of radioactive emissions, such as occur naturally in Cornwall and Scotland, and leukaemia. It is also known that clusters of leukaemia occur where there is no possible source of radioactivity.

Let us assume we have carried out a survey on the relationship between obesity and cancer. In the control group of 1,000 people, 10 were found to have developed cancer during the five years of the study, while 12 out of the 1,000 developed the disease in the obese group. One can see the headlines claiming that there is a 20 per cent greater risk of cancer if you are overweight. However, there is also evidence that fat people who develop cancer live longer than thin ones. As a result there will inevitably be more fat people alive with cancer than thin ones at any time, and this could account for these figures. To base government advice on this type of epidemiological evidence is dangerous. There are plenty of possible reasons why fat people have a slightly higher incidence of cancer than thin people, but the evidence that obesity *causes* cancer is weak.

It is an unfortunate product of information technology that it is increasingly easy to collect numbers. Numbers are used to determine policy, to reward effort and to condemn those not reaching targets. Nearly all of these numbers demonstrate a crude correlation between two events; they are, in fact, epidemiological studies. The government uses these fallible epidemiological statistics as though they were proven evidence. They are used to assess the achievement of education, policing, health policies and social behaviour. These raw statistics are meaningless unless and until they have been subject to corroboration by other means. To show that drinking red wine or eating vegetables is associated with a reduced incidence of cancer does not by itself prove that red wine and vegetables prevent cancer. It could be that those drinking the wine or eating the vegetables do not live long enough to suffer from the cancer! Casual associations of two events do not constitute proof. It is, at best, circumstantial evidence. It should not be used to infer that some schools achieve worse results than others, or some police forces arrest more criminals than others, or some food fads are healthy, unless there is other supporting evidence.

In this world of instant information, the validity of circumstantial evidence from the casual association of two events is too readily accepted as proof. Every day, the news media regale us with 'proof', nearly always based upon some epidemiological study, that this or that effect causes ill health. Often there is insufficient analysis of the way the information is collected and of the influence of factors that cannot be controlled, when the significance of the data is evaluated. We must recognise epidemiological surveys for what they are: circumstantial evidence that would not stand up in any court of law.

Chapter Four

THE HARM THAT PRESSURE GROUPS CAN DO

BY LORD TAVERNE

When Rachel Carson published *Silent Spring*, I fell under her spell. Her picture of a landscape devastated by pesticides, in which birds have vanished from the trees and fish from rivers, where flowers no longer blossom in the fields and people and animals die of mysterious diseases, was both moving and disturbing. She converted tens of thousands of people into passionate environmentalists and could fairly be called the mother of modern environmentalism. In the early 1970s, I joined Greenpeace and Friends of the Earth and read the works of Barry Commoner and Paul Ehrlich and *The Limits to Growth*, which persuaded me at the time not only that the natural world was being damaged almost beyond repair, but that the earth's resources would soon run out unless we abandoned our commitment to economic growth and ever-increasing consumption.

In one sense we are all environmentalists now, in that we regard the beauty of nature around us as one of the blessings in life and accept that we should not deprive our children and grandchildren of the enjoyment it gives us. But I am now a pragmatic environmentalist. I want to be sure that we do not base our actions on false fears and do not apply remedies which are unsupported by evidence and which do more harm than good. Gradually I came to realise that pressure groups that start out with the noblest intentions sometimes allow passion to overrule reason and the ends to corrupt the means. They can become casual about evidence and sometimes even deliberately mislead. They can become so obsessed with the need for publicity that, in the words of one of the world's best-known climate experts, Stephen Schneider 'to capture the public's imagination... we have to offer up scary scenarios, make simplified dramatic statements and make little mention of any doubts we have'. In fairness to Schneider, he continues by saying, 'Each of us has to decide the right balance between being effective and being honest. I hope that means doing both.' However, many environmentalists fail to balance risk against benefit; their actions often harm the causes they seek to promote.

Nearly all the forecasts of doom in *The Limits to Growth* turned out to be spectacularly wrong. They predicted that we would run out of gold, zinc, mercury and oil before 1992. Paul Ehrlich famously wrote: 'the battle to feed humanity is over. In the course of the 1970s hundreds of millions will starve to death.' (*The Population Bomb*, Ballantyne Books, 1968) Had we acted on these dire prophecies, the consequences would indeed have been disastrous. In Rachel Carson's case, the good she did in alerting us to the dangers of environmental degradation and the need to control the indiscriminate use of insecticides has been outweighed by the harm caused by a ban on DDT

DDT

Carson had some reason for warning the world about the dangers of DDT. There was evidence that it caused the thinning of eggshells with a possible effect on bird life, and its long-lasting properties coupled with its widespread use caused it to accumulate slowly in the food chain. It can still be detected in animals decades after spraying has ceased, and even in human breast milk, although it should be noted that present-day chemical tests can detect just one molecule in 1,000,000,000,000,000 (one in a million billion).

The evidence of a potential damage to wildlife might in itself have justified an end to its uncontrolled agricultural use. But Carson also forecast that DDT would be a cause of cancer and hepatitis, despite the fact that there has never been evidence of any harmful effects of DDT on human health. In the Second World War many people were exposed to high concentrations of DDT without any apparent ill effect. According to a report in 1971 by the National Academy of Sciences in the United States to advise the Environmental Protection Agency, 'The chronic toxicity studies on DDT have provided no indication that the insecticide is unsafe for humans'.

Against these potential dangers stands the devastating effect of banning the use of DDT: Carson didn't seem to take into account the vital role the insecticide played in controlling the transmission of malaria by killing the mosquitoes that carry the parasite. According to an earlier report by the US National Academy in 1970, in the two decades before DDT was banned it saved over 50 million lives. This view was endorsed by the World Health Organisation. It is the single most effective agent ever developed for saving human life. In Sri Lanka, for example, DDT reduced the number of cases of malaria in 1963 to 17; by 1968, after DDT was banned, the number of cases had risen to 2.5 million. A virtual ban on DDT has become effective in many parts of the world; as a result, malaria has come back with a vengeance. Over a million children in Africa die from it every year. Rachel Carson is a warning to us all of the dangers of neglecting the evidence-based approach and the need to weigh potential risk against benefit: it can be argued that the anti-DDT campaign she inspired was responsible for almost as many deaths as some of the worst dictators of the last century.

The campaign for a worldwide ban on DDT and other pesticides continues, although it is based on a different rationale. The World Wildlife Fund argues for a ban on the grounds that the pesticides are a hormone-disrupting chemical and may affect immune, reproductive and nervous systems in some animals. But arguments against retaining DDT for the spraying of the inside walls of houses are mistaken. Such spraying is the cheapest and still the most effective way of preventing malaria. There is no evidence that it presents any risk to humans. Any objective assessment of risks and benefits would come down firmly against a ban.

CAMPAIGNS BY GREENPEACE

The campaign against the use of DDT is a clear example of the harm produced by ignoring scientific evidence. The same can be said of some of the campaigns by Greenpeace and its allies. The history of the Brent Spar oil rig is a notorious case of the regard for evidence being sacrificed to the need to 'capture the public's imagination'.

In 1995, Shell decided to sink the giant Brent Spar oil rig in the deep Atlantic. After careful consultation it had concluded that this was the most environmentally friendly method of disposal, not least because the oceans are deficient in iron which is necessary for the growth of marine life. Greenpeace claimed that the rig was full of poisonous residues and that sinking it would pollute the ocean. Day after day brave Greenpeace eco-warriors in their small inflatables were shown on television harassing the giant tugs that towed the rig. Shell petrol stations were boycotted all over Europe until the oil company was forced to turn back the tugs and agree to dispose of the rig on dry land. It was a triumph for Greenpeace, the environmental David that had humbled the industrial Goliath.

In reality, the losers were not only Shell but also the environment. There were no poisonous residues in the rig – Greenpeace was eventually forced to apologise for its unfounded accusation – and so disposal on land was much less environmentally friendly than disposal in the ocean. Moreover, the pressure group could not have had total faith in its own propaganda: in 1986 its ship the *Rainbow Warrior*, which had been irreparably damaged by French saboteurs, was deliberately sunk off the New Zealand coast by Greenpeace, who claimed it would make a new reef highly beneficial to marine life.

Other Greenpeace campaigns also often damage the environment they claim to protect. Whenever a combined heat and power (CHP) plant is proposed as an efficient means of generating electricity, Greenpeace opposes it. Every incinerator, it claims, increases the amount of dioxins, invariably described as 'the most dangerous chemical known to man', in the air. When Greenpeace wins, the toxic waste is disposed of in landfill sites to which it normally has to be transported over long distances by lorry. Furthermore, the alternative to a CHP plant is invariably a less efficient form of energy generation that releases more greenhouse gases. The environment is more, not less, polluted. As for dioxins, not only do modern incinerators discharge only small amounts into the air, but their demonic properties are hugely exaggerated and largely spurious. The distinguished chemist John Emsley has pointed out that only four people, none of them members of the public, have ever been known to die of dioxin poisoning. The notorious accident at Seveso in 1976 released a massive amount of dioxins. This led to many cases of the skin condition chloracne, but no deaths. Too often environmentalists ignore the effect of the dose on toxicity – indeed, there is evidence that small doses of dioxins may be beneficial rather than harmful to human health.

GM CROPS

The issue that has in some ways become the crucial battlefield between belief in evidence and belief in dogma is the dispute about genetically modified crops. In many ways, the campaign against GM technology echoes the campaign against DDT. As argued in other essays in this volume, there is no evidence that GM crops have ever damaged human health, while they have already shown substantial benefits to some of the world's poorest farmers and can potentially make a huge contribution to the reduction of poverty, hunger and disease. Over five million small farmers in China, India, South Africa and elsewhere now farm GM cotton. Not only has their income been substantially increased by savings from the reduced use of pesticides, but their health has also improved. These are actual, proven benefits.

However, the most important feature of genetic modification is its potential: crops can be genetically modified to grow in arid or saline regions where no crops can grow today; staple crops can be protected against diseases that destroy small farmers' livelihoods; vaccines from plants can offer protection against hepatitis B and childhood diarrhoea that causes millions of deaths. None of these is yet in production, although the technology exists.

There have been plenty of scare stories about GM products. The one that led to fears about 'Frankenstein food' arose from an experiment by Arpad Pusztai who claimed that some genetically modified potatoes damaged the immune system of rats. His findings, which were broadcast on television before they had been scientifically evaluated, were carefully examined by a Royal Society committee and utterly discredited. There is no reason to regard GM crops as less safe for human consumption than conventional crops: this is the opinion of three other Royal Society reports, one report by seven international academies of sciences, as well as any number of reports by other prestigious committees, including two by the Nuffield Council on Bioethics (a mixed committee of scientific experts and lay representatives). Nor has any evidence emerged that they will create new 'super-weeds' or that they are especially dangerous to biodiversity.

The most notorious misinformation about the damage they cause to the environment concerned a laboratory study on the monarch butterfly. However, the experiment was later shown to be deeply flawed. Field tests, as opposed to the laboratory study, showed that the impact on the butterflies of pollen from GM corn was no different from the effects of conventional corn.

Nevertheless, the literature produced by environmental activists constantly refers to the danger to human health from GM crops 'as proved by Dr Pusztai', the threat that they will give rise to 'super-weeds' by cross-pollination and the harm they have caused to monarch butterflies. So effective is the propaganda by green non-government organisations (NGOs) that in 2003 the Zambian government refused food aid from America because, according to a government spokesman, 'We would rather let our people starve than feed them toxic food.' China, which leads the world in applying GM technology to crops that are the staple foods of poor countries, is now hesitant about granting licences for the commercial cultivation of GM crops because of fears for its exports.

Several well-known aid agencies, widely respected for their dedication to the cause of reducing hunger, poverty and disease, are prominent in the anti-GM campaign. It is difficult to explain their paradoxical alliance with green NGOs like Greenpeace and Friends of the Earth. Some of the aid agencies and green NGOs seem to have formed an esoteric club in which they perpetuate each other's prejudices without any contact with experts outside their own ranks. I have talked to two aid agencies that have made public pronouncements about the dangerous nature of GM crops without any contact with expert plant biologists.

One explanation of this stance is a shared hostility to multinational companies that have developed GM crops. They suspect them of sinister motives because they do not believe companies should pursue profits while they themselves are selflessly dedicated to the service of mankind. But whatever the reasons, a lack of respect for evidence and an almost religious belief that GM crops are dangerous leads to paradoxical results.

For example, a document produced by ActionAid, 'Going Against the Grain', ridicules the potential of 'golden rice'. This is rice genetically modified to induce it to synthesise a precursor that is converted into vitamin A in the body. Outside green NGO circles, it has been widely hailed as a development of enormous potential for good because it can help to supplement diets deficient in vitamin A that are a major cause of blindness and child mortality in developing countries. However, 'Against the Grain' quotes a study by Greenpeace, which has not been published in any peer-reviewed journals, that states that a child would have to eat seven kilograms of rice a day to benefit from it. The scientists who developed golden rice have demonstrated that this overstates the amount children would have to eat by more than 15 times since golden rice is designed to act as a supplement to vitamin A deficiency and not to supply all the vitamin A children need. But ActionAid and Greenpeace are not, it seems, swayed by evidence or balance. None of the weighty studies by the top scientific academies, including those of India, China, Brazil, Mexico and the Academy of Sciences for the Developing World, is quoted in the ActionAid report. Instead, it relies almost entirely on information from green pressure groups.

The same anti-GM lobbies that persuaded Zambia to choose starvation rather than food aid from America may well succeed in delaying the introduction of golden rice. As a result, more children will go blind. As a study by the Nuffield Council on Bioethics observed, we have a moral duty to make the potential benefits of GM technology available to the developing world.

AIDS

Another example of the disastrous effects of rejecting scientific evidence relates to AIDS in South Africa. In this case the blame does not lie directly with pressure groups, but is related to mistrust of multinational companies which has been nurtured by NGOs (although companies themselves are not free from blame). President Thabo Mbeki espoused the iconoclastic views of the maverick Dr Peter Duesberg that AIDS is not associated with HIV and cannot be prevented or treated by anti-retroviral drugs. The South African government claimed that anti-HIV drugs were an attempt to commit the genocide of black people and that retrovirals were akin to 'the biological warfare of the apartheid era'. President Mbeki favoured a return to traditional African remedies. As a result many people died whose deaths might have been prevented.

THE BACK-TO-NATURE CULT

The South African AIDS disaster raises a wider question: is there any connection between the anti-DDT campaign, hostility to GM crops, a general unfounded fear of chemicals and the rejection of Western medicine? I believe there is. They are all part of a back-to-nature, nature-knows-best approach that essentially rejects the scientific revolution that was part of the Enlightenment. Rachel Carson regarded science and technology as dangerous because they arose from mankind's mistaken attempt to control nature. The predecessors of the present-day environmentalists saw science as 'a mechanistic, rapacious, inorganic attitude towards nature'. Critics of GM crops are particularly disturbed because the technology can transfer genes between species and even between plants and animals, which is regarded as akin to 'playing God'. (They do not seem to object to the same technology being used to transfer genes from human beings into bacteria or yeasts in order to help people control their diabetes.)

The fashion for alternative medicine and traditional remedies, carried to extremes by Mbeki in his opposition to anti-retroviral drugs, is also based on the belief that practices based on nature are superior to modern medicine. The campaign against the mumps, measles and rubella triple vaccine (MMR) was led by JABS, a group of people who were ideologically opposed to vaccination. People forget that in the days before modern medicine life was nasty, brutish and short, and life expectancy was curtailed by the ravages of lethal infectious diseases which scientific medicine can now prevent or cure.

The rise in popularity of organic farming is another manifestation of the rejection of scientific evidence in favour of a mystical belief in 'nature'. Its principles are partly based on a belief that natural chemicals are good while synthetic ones are bad, ignoring the fact that numerous natural substances, ranging from arsenic to ricin and aflatoxin, are deadly poisons and many synthetic chemicals , such as anti-bacterial drugs, are beneficial. None of the claims made for organic produce has ever been upheld when tested. The Soil Association does claim to promote responsible animal husbandary and that is good news for animals. However, the Advertising Standards Association has twice made them withdraw leaflets making claims exclusively for organic farmers in this area. In response, Patrick Holden, President of the Soil Association, told the House of Lords select committee that science was not sufficiently developed to be able to measure the special qualities of organic farming. It seems to suggest that a belief in mysticism is necessary to appreciate organic food's 'special qualities'.

Indeed, organic is ultimately harmful because of its inherent inefficiency. Overall its yields are some 20–50 per cent lower than those of conventional farming. This is why organic produce costs more. Lower-income families who are persuaded by the constant propaganda that organic food is healthier will not buy cheaper conventional food. But if they pay higher prices for organic food they will be likely to spend less on fruit and vegetables that they need for a balanced diet. If the powerful organic-farming lobby succeeds in spreading its practices to the Third World, they would gravely aggravate the severe shortage of good farming land. Inefficient organic farming can offer no help to poor farmers in Africa in eliminating the pests and diseases that destroy half their produce. Yet the organic movement have made many statements and issued several pamphlets claiming that organic farming is the answer to the needs of the developing world. It is one of their most dangerous claims.

DISTORTING THE LANGUAGE

Yet the back-to-nature movement gets an immense coverage in the media. It challenges the scientific establishment. It is associated with a cause – saving the planet – about which everybody cares. It is promoted by a group of NGOs who are such past masters at public relations that they have even imposed their own terminology. The term 'Frankenfoods' was a brilliant invention. So was the phrase 'terminator seeds', used to describe seeds whose plants are sterile. The original purpose of 'terminator seeds' was an answer to the fears that cross-pollination would lead to 'contanimation'. This virtue was deliberately ignored by the anti-GM lobby. They argue that the seeds force farmers to buy new seeds every year. No doubt firms like Monsanto see this as a useful side-effect. As a result of the campaign against them, 'terminator' seeds were never marketed, although recently English Nature suggested that 'genetic incompatibility' should be engineered into crops – in other words that 'terminator seeds' should be developed after all.

The word 'contamination' is constantly used with reference to GM crops. 'Contamination' is used to refer to cross-pollination, a process familiar in nature. The flow of genes between related species, and occasionally across species barriers, is the reason for our planet's biodiversity. But 'contamination' implies corruption, pollution and impurity. The danger of GM 'contamination' is in fact another scare used to frighten us. When pejorative language is used for propaganda purposes, democrats should beware.

GOOD INTENTIONS AND GOOD SCIENCE

The examples I have cited show that good intentions are no guarantee of public benefit. Indeed, it is a common error to assume that what matters is motive, not results. We are told by the George Monbiots and other self-appointed guardians of our conscience who see capitalist conspiracies everywhere that anyone with any association with the corporate world cannot contribute to impartial debate or the welfare of mankind, because association with the profit motive corrupts integrity. Given that, regrettably, public investment in scientific research has declined and that most scientific and technological innovation depends on corporate funds, it follows that we should be suspicious of virtually all modern technology, from the washing machine to the computer.

In fact, though scientists have values, science does not. Science itself is objective, and, in evaluating the importance of scientific findings, the motives of the researcher are in the end irrelevant. What matters is the quality of the findings. Are they reproducible? Do they stand up to criticism? Researchers working for a company that makes a profit may also be concerned to benefit mankind. They can produce science which is as valid as researchers working for Greenpeace who may be motivated by a wish to gain publicity as well

– no doubt to preserve our environment. Conversely, the most public-spirited, completely independent scientists can produce bad science. In the end, the progress of science depends on evidence. Many NGOs promote many excellent causes, but, because too many of them do not regard respect for evidence as the golden rule, their actions often severely damage the causes they profess to serve.

PART TWO:

THE FOOD
WE EAT

Chapter Five

HEALTHY EATING

BY VINCENT MARKS

Good health is at the top of everyone's wish list – but what is it? Although we know if we are unwell, there is no completely satisfactory way of knowing if we are in good health.

A dictionary definition of health – 'soundness of body: that condition in which its functions are duly and efficiently discharged' – says nothing about future expectations. Longevity is almost as important as good health, and the two are not synonymous, as evidenced by the life histories of Florence Nightingale and Charles Darwin: both suffered ill health for much of their very long lives. Nor has good health much to do with 'fitness'. There are too many reported incidents of athletes dropping down dead at the height of their powers, and of longevity in the sedentary, to support such a connection.

A more useful definition is the absence of discomfort, illness or disease or the imminent expectation of it. This is the logic behind screening patients with the aim of finding people with curable diseases such as TB before they cause irrevocable damage.

While proper nutrition does not ensure perfect health, it is a prerequisite for it. Until comparatively recently, proper nutrition was only available to the affluent, rich and powerful. The situation changed with the advances in the science and technology of food production, preservation and transportation made during the late nineteenth and early twentieth centuries, and with our increased understanding of the science of nutrition. This has made it possible to provide most people, especially those living in what is quaintly described as the developed world, with a plentiful supply – some would say too plentiful a supply – of wholesome food.

Why, then, are newspapers, television and radio so obsessed with what we eat? They claim that our nutrition is so poor that we are in danger of reversing the enormous improvements we saw during the twentieth century. If this is so, it is certainly not due to a lack of advice. However, once one starts to question the soundness of that advice and where it comes from, one begins to understand the nature of the problem.

Improvements in public health during the first half of the twentieth century made great strides in reducing premature deaths from infections, industrial hazards and the major nutritional diseases. This led to the unrealistic belief that all illnesses, except congenital ones, are preventable if only their cause was known. Although the germ theory of disease explained and helped to eliminate many of the commonest illnesses in the past, it did little to help us understand the chronic illnesses that afflict the middle-aged and elderly. More recently, it has been realised that most chronic illnesses are the result of the interplay between a person's genetic make-up and the way they live. What and how much they eat is possibly the most important environmental factor in the causation of chronic illness.

Myocardial infarction – an acute heart attack caused by coronary thrombosis – was rare at the start of the twentieth century, but by the 1960s it was the commonest cause of death in many of the countries of the developed world, including the UK. This was labelled a disease of affluence in spite of the fact that it was more common among the poor. Epidemiological studies suggested that both genetic and environmental factors were implicated in its causation. In some families, the genetic link was direct and very obvious from one generation to the next, but in most cases the link was tenuous or non-existent.

Lung cancer, on the other hand, whose rise in incidence was almost as rapid and catastrophic, seemed to have no genetic basis, and it was Richard Doll, using epidemiological methods, who laid it squarely at the door of cigarette smoking. Doll went on to establish that people who voluntarily gave up smoking reduced, although they did not abolish, their risk of developing lung cancer. Put differently, a model epidemiological study pointed the finger of blame at cigarette smoking, but it was the interventional studies that established the causal link between smoking and disease. This level of evidence has rarely been repeated – particularly in relation to diet where, with few exceptions, the results of interventional studies have been disappointing. This may be because, while eating is obligatory, smoking is not.

The quality of evidence linking diet to specific diseases is poor, apart from common 'simple deficiency diseases' such as scurvy (vitamin C deficiency), rickets (vitamin D deficiency), anaemia (iron deficiency) and protein-calorie malnutrition. The evidence is usually unconvincing, contradictory and almost impossible to confirm experimentally.

Food habits, including portion size, are acquired at a very early age, mostly from parents but also, to a lesser extent, from one's peers. They can be extremely difficult to change even when the motivation for doing so is great. This may be why, despite a plethora of reports suggesting the benefits of this or that diet, they have so little effect. The evidence that they do any good, except in the grossly malnourished, is very shaky. This is in contrast to the obvious benefits of sound nutritional advice and the provision of nutritious food during the first half of the twentieth century. This was the time when the science of human nutrition can be considered to have become established. Nutrition is therefore a comparatively new science, involving the study of the interactions between a person and their food and drink. This distinguishes it from dietetics, which is about the use of foods to attempt to treat or prevent disease, and catering and food science, both of which are professions in their own right.

Human nutrition is less well developed as a science than animal nutrition, which is driven by commercial agricultural interests and has the great advantage that it is amenable to experimental study and evaluation. Animal nutritionists can specify the chemical composition of diets, and the amounts to be fed, how often and at what times of the day in order to produce the desired effect in any particular breed of animals or birds. By the addition of lysine, an essential amino acid in short supply in many vegetables, it is possible, for example, to accelerate the growth of piglets in order to bring them to market earlier, producing a significant cost saving. Despite all their best endeavours, however, animal nutritionists do not always get it right. They knew that when cows gave higher yields of milk they lost too much protein. To overcome this problem they fed them high-quality animal proteins, but it was not until it was too late that it was found that this could disseminate the 'mad cow disease' BSE.

While many of the lessons learned from animal nutrition, including those conducted on experimental laboratory animals in the course of clinical research, are applicable to man, they can, at best, only point us in the right direction. They do not permit definitive conclusions, as the differences in the metabolic requirements are greater between species than within them. This obvious fact does not prevent the headline writers from proclaiming the result of some research project to be a great advance in nutrition, without pointing out that it was only found in one breed of a particular species and not likely to be reproducible in humans.

The pioneers of both animal and human nutrition were concerned with the chemical composition both of the body and of food, and how one was transformed into the other. They started with our understanding of the nature and structure of proteins, the role of carbohydrates and fats as sources of energy and the need for various mineral elements such as sodium, calcium and iodine. Knowledge of the vital role played by vitamins came much later, and did not reach its zenith until the early to mid-twentieth century, when vitamin B12, the last vitamin to be named, was isolated.

Sir Robert McCarrison, in a landmark series of lectures entitled 'Nutrition and National Health' published in 1936, said, 'Man is made up of what he eats.' This statement is of course true, whereas the phrase 'you are what you eat', often found in articles written for the lay public by people calling themselves 'nutritionists', is patently rubbish. McCarrison, an observational and experimental nutritionist of the highest calibre, differentiated good from bad diets. Poor diets, he believed, were commonplace in Britain and responsible for much of the chronic illness suffered by the working class. Iron-deficiency anaemia, for example, was rife among women. In 1936, no less than 52 per cent of men presenting themselves to army recruiting offices in the UK, and 68 per cent of those from the large conurbations, were rejected by the military on health grounds due to their poor nutritional status.

McCarrison advocated a diet providing whole cereal grains, milk and milk products such as butter and cheese, pulses, vegetables and occasional meat. He was also in favour of supplementing foods with minerals, such as iron, iodine and calcium, and vitamins which, during the Second World War when traditional foods were in short supply, were seldom present in sufficient quantities in the diets of either the well-to-do or the poor. Rationing, because it made food of suitable quality and affordable prices available to everyone, undoubtedly improved the nutritional status of the population as a whole. Since that time we have never looked back – although you would not think so from the flood of dietary advice that emanates from individuals and official and quasi-official committees, and which fills our newspapers, magazines, radios and television channels.

Disease attributable to poor-quality food is fortunately largely a thing of the past in the developed world. It has to some extent been replaced by anxiety about the effects of overindulgence in energy-rich foods. Less well-recognised is undernutrition, which is most common in the elderly, especially the sick. They are not helped by being fed a supposedly healthy 'low energy-dense' diet when they are in a hospital or nursing home because it is 'politically correct' to do so.

What they need is lots of high-energy food that is palatable and which they can enjoy. This often means a diet that is rich in sugar and fat. Dairy ice cream, for example, can be made to incorporate all of the essential minerals and vitamins, and is usually appreciated even by the most fastidious of eaters.

There has probably never been a shortage of individuals or committees prepared to offer advice on how to improve one's own health, but the idea of improving the health of the nation by dietary means is comparatively new. The McGovern Senate Committee in America, which set dietary goals for the USA in February 1977, was probably the first to have governmental backing. By 1988, the European office of WHO could refer to 18 sets of recommendations for dietary changes that might reduce the incidence of diseases common in middle life. Advice to reduce fat intake, increase complex carbohydrate intake and reduce salt and sugar intake was a frequent theme. It came about largely by the selection of committee members who believed in this particular mantra, and the selective citing of research papers to reflect their collective preconceptions while they ignored those that did not.

Catchphrases and jingles, especially those with an emotive message, are easy to remember. Consequently it is simpler to talk of 'safety' and 'toxicity' as though they are absolutes and opposites, rather than merely a reflection of the dose of the same substance. Many nutrients, especially minerals and vitamins, are toxic when used in excess, but clearly essential and, therefore, safe when used properly. But individuals differ in their requirements. Failure to recognise this simple, obvious fact accounts for a number of hospital admissions each year by people who believe that if a little is 'good' then more must be better. While this attitude has taught us much about the effects of gross dietary indiscretions, we are still abysmally ignorant of the adverse effects of modest but prolonged underprovision or overusage of essential nutrients, as well as other inappropriate eating patterns. The truth is that we know remarkably little about the long-term effects of dietary changes – not only in the chemical composition of food, but also in the way we prepare and eat it. To suggest, as is fashionable, that traditional methods of preparing food are safer and better than the current industrial methods used for prepared or oven-ready food is not based on fact but on surmise and prejudice.

Through food science, we have a wealth of knowledge about what different methods of food preparation and storage do to its composition and texture. This is the reason why we now have not only 'use by' but also 'best by' dates on all prepared foods. The growth of consumerism – albeit frequently misguided and often based upon false logic rather than genuine knowledge – has, within the past couple of decades, brought home the cost of our lack of knowledge of human nutrition. In the land of the blind, the one-eyed man is king: consequently, many people with a smattering of knowledge and a familiarity with the terminology claim to be experts. This, when combined with an ability to wield a pen, write persuasively and project oneself well on radio and television, produces a limitless opportunity to propagate unproven and irrational beliefs.

The increase in the number of instant experts needed to fill the acres of vacant newspaper pages has coincided with the rise of paternalism and authoritarianism among a vociferous group of individuals, some of them extremely knowledgeable and sincere, who argue that the public should be told what is and is not 'good for them' on the basis of their interpretation of the published data. Such individuals may call themselves 'health educators', but they are really propagandists. They may have enjoyed some justifiable successes, such as the requirement for more informative food labelling – but that in itself is contentious. Exactly what information and how much of it a label could and should contain is open to debate. Differentiating sugars into 'natural' or 'added', for example, is nonsensical, as is the differentiation of food into organic and, I suppose by inference, 'inorganic', rather than differentiation according to its freshness and nutritive value.

To be effective, food labelling must not only be within the law but also intellectually honest. It is common, for example, to see products from reputable manufacturers that claim to contain 'no added sugars' when they are already so full of sugar that any addition would make the product unpalatable. Fruit juices and baked beans sweetened with concentrated apple juice are examples that spring to mind. One might as well sell gin labelled 'no added alcohol' as fruit juice labelled 'no added sugar'.

The average health and longevity of the population in Britain has never been better – despite the increase in the prevalence of obesity and the illnesses that it causes. Much of this is undoubtedly due to the availability of wholesome food whose quality is assured by rigorous monitoring and which is sold at a price that most people can afford. While the food industry can be justifiably proud of its contribution to this improvement in nutritional status, it can also be castigated for promoting its products with advertisements that, although not untrue, do mislead by implication. But the same charge can be levied at the food propagandists who make their living and reputations by vilifying the food industry for using improper but legitimate means, within the current commercial climate, to persuade people to buy their products.

In order to improve the health of the nation through dietary means, it is necessary to ensure that health education is firmly based on the science of nutrition. This requires a basic knowledge of food preparation and presentation, of cooking and catering, as well as an understanding of physiology and metabolism – all of which should be taught as core subjects at school. Only then will children, when they grow up, be able to choose the most appropriate foods to eat and not be misled by ambiguous or deliberately slanted messages from commercial or governmental sources that are fashionable but not necessarily correct. The famous food pyramid, introduced to simplify the healthy eating message and based upon 1980s dogma, is already outmoded and incorrect. What is the best advice on healthy eating today? I believe that, as in the past, we should eat a variety of different foods from the dairy, grocer, baker, fruiterer, greengrocer and vintner, and somewhat less frequently from the fishmonger and butcher, in portion sizes and total quantity that ensures proper growth in children and the maintenance of a body mass index of around 20–25 in young adults and 23–27 in older adults. This, coupled with moderate daily exercise, involves a lifestyle that becomes easier to practise once one understands the reason why it is good for one's health.

Chapter Six

OBESITY

BY VINCENT MARKS

'Corpulence in America is regarded, along with narcotic addiction, as something wicked, and I shall not be surprised if soon we have a prohibition against it in the name of national security.'

ASTWOOD, 1962

The Myth: **Obesity is caused by eating the 'wrong kinds of food'.**
The Fact: **The most likely causes of obesity in humans are hormonal and genetic.**

Obesity has always been with us but, whereas in the past it was the prerogative of the rich, it is now the scourge of the poor. We are told by numerous newspaper articles, life-insurance companies' publicity material and governmental publications that it has reached 'epidemic proportions'. It is blamed on 'junk food', but the real reason for its increasing incidence is far more complicated.

Obesity develops when energy intake exceeds energy expenditure. It will be maintained until this balance is reversed. The supply of food as well as the type of food is involved from the start. Until recently, food was only plentiful for the rich – the poor often lived at subsistence level, although they frequently performed more manual work over longer periods. The ability to get fat was a status symbol, and still is in some parts of the world. Although now looked upon as a hazard to health, the ability to become fat in times when food was not constantly available could have had an important survival value in the past. People who were fat at the start of a famine would have a better chance of surviving than those who were thin. Being fat has become a cosmetic problem for the fashion-conscious over the last half-century, and it is the social desirability of being thin that produces the huge diet and weight-reduction industry. The medical problems caused by obesity, however, have only been recognised more recently. Should we worry about getting fat? Yes, because in the long term it predisposes us to a variety of illnesses and a shortened life expectancy, even though some fat people live their full three score years and ten and more.

Until about 20 years ago, though, the term 'overweight' was applied to those who exceeded the ideal weight used by the Metropolitan Life Assurance Company, and whose tables adorned most commercial weighing scales, now largely discarded. A new way of expressing fatness has gained ground more recently, making for ease of communication and epidemiological studies. The body mass index, or BMI, relates weight to height through a formula devised in the nineteenth century by a Belgian epidemiologist, Adolph Quetelet. A person's BMI is their weight in kilograms divided by the square of their height in metres. Although it has shortcomings – it says nothing about the proportion of body weight that is fat, which is the real test of obesity – the BMI has become the recognised standard of measurement for fatness.

Most healthy young adults have a BMI of 20–25. Those with a BMI less than 20 are classified as underweight and those with a BMI of 25–30 as overweight or plump. A BMI of over 30 is arbitrarily classified as indicating obesity. Insurance company statistics reveal that people with BMIs under 20 or over 30 are poorer life risks than those with BMIs between 20 and 30. As people get older, there is population shift from the lower to the upper half of this range. Plumpness in late-middle and old age, especially in women, is not as great a health risk as it is in young and middle-aged adults – indeed it is an advantage for longevity. Plumpness in childhood, often called 'puppy fat', is common, and the evidence linking it to adult obesity is conflicting. What is certain, though, is that gross obesity is a real hazard but, in spite of what one reads in the media, this is rare and normally due to genetic and metabolic defects. It is a medical problem from the start.

Fat constitutes a higher proportion of a woman's body weight than a man's. It is only when fat deposits become abnormally large – which can be difficult to determine simply by measuring weight alone – that it becomes appropriate to talk of obesity. There are almost as many types of obesity as there are individuals afflicted by it. However, two main physical types can usually be distinguished.

Gynaecoid obesity, so called because it is more common in women, is associated with increased deposition of fat in and under the skin – especially below the waist – and is relatively benign. Android obesity, on the other hand, is much more malign. It is more common in men and is due to massive deposition of fat within the abdominal cavity. It gives rise to what is often, but wrongly, described as a beer belly. People, including women, with this type of truncal obesity have larger waist than hip measurements, and their limbs are often surprisingly thin. They are sometimes described as apples in contrast to the fancifully described pear shape of those with gynaecoid obesity. When associated with certain biochemical abnormalities and/or high blood pressure, people with truncal obesity are said to have the 'metabolic syndrome'. It is the catastrophic rise in prevalence of this condition, rather than of fatness, that is the major cause for concern. Neither type of obesity is an illness in its own right, but each predisposes to the development of incapacity or premature death. Diseases such as diabetes and coronary heart disease are much commoner in people with the metabolic syndrome.

Like all conditions from which mankind suffers, obesity is the result of the interplay between nature, in the shape of genetic and antenatal factors, and nurture, principally in the shape of the availability of food. While this may seem obvious, it has not always been accepted. As recently as the beginning of the twentieth century, the link between food intake and obesity was appreciated by very few. Anecdotal personal experience suggested that fat people ate no more than thin ones – some of whom seemed to be bottomless pits into which food could be shovelled with seemingly little effect. There is no doubt that this perception is wrong. Statistically, fat people both expend and consume more calories than thin people, although the overlap between them is enormous. This is mainly due to differences in resting metabolism – the amount of energy required just to keep body warm – and the levels of physical activity or exercise. It is quite easy to show mathematically that quite subtle differences in food intake or energy expenditure could, over a period of many years, produce profound changes in body shape. For example, taking in the energy contained in just one knifeful of butter more than you expend every day would, after a year, theoretically cause a two-kilogram gain in weight.

This simplistic approach to the causes of obesity belies its complexity. What is truly remarkable is how most people manage to maintain a more or less constant weight once they reach adulthood without a conscious effort to control what they eat. It is as if they possessed a 'bodystat' analogous to a thermostat in a refrigerator. The mechanics of this bodystat are still being unravelled by biochemists and physiologists throughout the world, and by psychologists, sociologists and epidemiologists in individual communities. The role of nature – genetics – rather than nurture in the process of getting fat has been known to farmers, veterinarians and experimentalists for over a hundred years, but was only recently established in human beings. This began with studies of the differences in the incidence of obesity in identical and non-identical twins brought up separately from one another. Identical twins looked and weighed the same: non-identical ones didn't.

Gross obesity occurs in several very inbred strains of rodents. In one strain, the specific gene responsible was given the name ob for obesity. Mice inheriting a copy of the gene from both parents develop a condition that lead to them depositing so much fat that they weighed four to five times as much as their siblings who did not have the gene or had inherited just one copy of it. The fat ones lacked the ability to make a hormone called leptin which, among its many properties, has the ability to suppress appetite. ob/ob mice eat ravenously until they are so fat they cannot get to their food. Even when fed only as much as their thin siblings, they still put on more weight. Within the past 10 years, a similar condition has been recognised in human beings, although it is extremely rare. Another genetic type of obesity in mice causes a condition that resembles ob/ob, but is caused by an inability to respond to leptin.

The idea that hormones played a part in controlling body weight began with the discovery that patients with thyrotoxicosis, caused by an overactive thyroid gland, often develop ravenous appetites yet lose weight. Conversely, those with an underactive thyroid often gain weight, though they very rarely become obese. Investigations into the role of the thyroid gland showed it played no part in the genesis of obesity. It has only been since the discovery of leptin and several other hormones that are concerned with the control of appetite that interest in the place of hormones has been rekindled.

Unfortunately, we still have a long way to go in understanding how these more recently discovered hormones work. Contrary to expectations, most fat people have more leptin in their blood than normal, so treatment by giving them leptin is unlikely to work. Equally exciting is the discovery that at least two other hormones, both produced in the intestines in response to certain foods, affect the metabolism of the body. Genetically engineered animals, rendered insensitive to a hormone called GIP, do not become obese with overfeeding. This supports earlier work, derived from studies in human beings, which suggests that GIP is one of the factors that lead to people becoming obese.

Contrary to popular belief, it is extremely difficult to become clinically obese by voluntarily eating excessively. This was established by experiments performed on healthy young volunteer prisoners. These experiments showed that mere access to unlimited supplies of food was not enough for the average person to become obese: something more was required. It clearly has something to do with appetite and the ability to overcome the feeling of satiety that most people experience when they have eaten sufficient for their physical requirements. A recently discovered hormone produced in the intestine called PYY works on the brain to suppress appetite. Under experimental conditions, it enables obese people to resist the temptation to eat excessively. It is currently being pursued as a potential treatment for obesity. Other gut hormones affecting appetite and the sense of satiety have also been discovered. One of these is GLP-1. Like GIP and PYY, it is made and released from the intestine in response to certain foods; like GIP, it is involved with the disposition of the individual constituents of the food within the body, mainly – though not exclusively – through their ability to stimulate the release of insulin. How important these and many other newly discovered hormones are in the genesis of obesity awaits further studies. It is one thing to discover an active chemical in inbred rodents or individual human beings under research conditions, but quite another to apply it in clinical conditions.

While the availability of a plentiful supply of food is a prerequisite for the development of obesity, the relationship is far from being a simple one. Just as most people with access to alcohol do not become alcoholics, a few, especially those with a genetic predisposition, do. But whereas it is possible to abstain from alcohol completely – and so achieve a cure of the ill – this option is not available to the obese.

The idea currently being propagated by single-issue pressure groups that obesity is due to one particular type of food constituent whether it be fat, sugar, rapidly absorbed starches or combinations of them – in particular, when they are provided in the form of foods such as hamburgers, pizzas, chips, crisps and other energy-rich nibbles – would be laughable if it were not so misleading. Obesity is a genuine recognisable medical problem. It will not be resolved by simplistic dogma that is based on unproven opinion rather than on evidence.

The fact that an increase in the incidence of obesity coincided with a rise in the availability of fast foods is not evidence of their role in its causation. Exactly the same argument could be advanced for the rise in central heating. Human beings burn off many more calories to stay alive in a cold environment than when they are warm. It would nevertheless be as foolish to assume that the answer to obesity is to return to the days of cold and damp housing as it is to suggest that banning the sale of energy-dense fast foods will solve the problem. Decades of dietary advice for the prevention and treatment of obesity based on avoiding first this and then that type of food have all resulted in failure. Any new way of losing weight is likely to produce an effect lasting a year or two, especially if aided by pharmaceutical appetite suppressants. A small percentage of dieters do manage to sustain their weight loss, but this is achieved not merely by changes in their diet but also by altering their whole way of life. Indeed, the few long-term, large-scale interventional studies that have succeeded in reducing the incidence of obesity, and more especially type-2 diabetes, have relied upon intensive re-education and alterations in lifestyle to incorporate changes in exercise as well as in eating habits.

The way food is eaten, whether as regular meals or 'on the hoof', the time of eating, the size of individual portions and what they consist of as well as the genetic and hormonal factors in the person eating the food all have a part to play. The old adage that it is better to leave the dining table wanting more than to leave it fully satiated is probably still as good advice as any for those genuinely wanting to avoid obesity. This may be difficult to achieve in an 'I want it now' society, but it might be helped by teaching nutrition and the long-term health risks of obesity at an early age rather than resorting to propaganda based on half-truths and unproven ideas.

But for many of the morbidly obese, the ones really at risk, it is only advances in the understanding of the pathology of obesity and its specific and appropriate treatment that offer any genuine hope of sustained benefit.

Chapter Seven

JUNK FOOD

BY STANLEY FELDMAN

The Myth: **A salad is better for you than a Big Mac.**

The Fact: **Many prepacked salads have more calories than a Big Mac.**

The term 'junk food' is an oxymoron. Either something is a food, in which case it is not junk, or it has no nutritional value, in which case it cannot be called a food. It can't be both. Ask most people what they understand by the term and they think of McDonald's hamburgers. None of their explanations for why hamburgers are junk food makes any sense; rather, they believe hamburgers are the cause of serious health problems because they have been told it is so.

Some rather ill-informed individuals have so convinced themselves of the dangers of hamburgers that they have suggested taxing them. Quite why hamburgers should be considered such a threat to our health that they should be singled out for taxation defies reason. Why should mincing a piece of beef turn it from being a 'good food' into one that is such dangerous 'junk' that it needs to be taxed in order to dissuade people from eating it? What would happen if, instead of mincing the meat, it was chopped into chunks and made into boeuf bourguignon – should it be taxed at only 50 per cent? To try to justify this illogical proposal, these self-appointed food experts tell us that hamburgers contain more fat than a fillet steak. They fail to point out that the ratio of protein to fat in a hamburger is usually higher than in most lamb chops, and that most hamburgers contain less fat than a Sainsbury's Waldorf salad.

But, that aside, why should the fat be bad? Would these same people like to tax the cheese offered at the end of the meal because, after all, it contains the same basic animal fat as the hamburger? Or perhaps it is the hamburger bun that they feel is unhealthy. But the same self-appointed dietary experts would not object to a helping of food in the form of pasta or a slice or two of wholemeal brown bread (which, by the way, is the bread with the highest level of pesticide). The pasta, the bread and the bun produce a similar carbohydrate load in our food and are absorbed into the bloodstream as the same constituents. As for the tomato ketchup on the hamburger, it is rich in vitamin C and the antioxidant polyphenols that are supposed to keep cell degeneration and cancer at bay.

There is no such thing as junk food. All food is composed of carbohydrate, fat and protein. An intake of a certain amount of each is essential for a healthy life. In addition, a supply of certain minerals, such as iron, calcium and tiny amounts of selenium, and a supply of vitamins, fibre, salt and fluid contribute to health. Once the necessary amounts of carbohydrate, fat and protein have been taken, any long-term surplus is stored as glycogen or fat in the body. Protein is protein whether it comes from an Aberdeen Angus steak or a McDonald's hamburger. It is broken up in the gut into its amino-acid building blocks, which are identical in both the hamburger and the steak; and although the relative amounts of each particular amino acid may vary slightly, this has no nutritional significance. These broken-down products of protein are absorbed into the bloodstream to be restructured into body proteins in the various cells of the body. Any excess ends up as fat. One source of animal protein is not necessarily of better value to the body than another, nor is it more or less fattening. A diet consisting only of Aberdeen Angus steak would be as 'junky' as one composed only of hamburgers. Similarly, animal fat is broken down and absorbed in the same way whether it originated in a hamburger, a lamb chop or the cheese on top of a pasta dish.

We need some fat in our diet, not only because it contains essential fat-soluble vitamins but also because it contributes much of the taste to foods. Very lean meat is tasteless unless enriched by a sauce containing fatty flavouring. No one would suggest that eating hamburgers and chips every day would constitute a good diet, but it would be better than one made up of Waldorf salad. The answer lies in a diet that is both varied and balanced.

We have been so indoctrinated about the evils of junk food, a concept so closely tied up with hamburgers that, if you were to ask the man in the street which was the better meal, pâté de foie gras or a hamburger, he would almost certainly condemn the hamburger. In terms of its contribution to the food requirements of the body, the pâté, with its high cholesterol and fat and low-value protein, approaches the junk-food profile while a hamburger with tomato ketchup has good mixed-food value. A tomato, basil and chicken salad from Safeway is presented as 'healthy food' although it contains roughly the same amount of fat and calories as a Big Mac and chips (*Sunday Times*, August 2004). If, instead of eating a Big Mac, people were suddenly to start eating these salads, it is unlikely they would be any healthier or lose any weight.

There is no doubt that snobbery and cost contributes to the perception of what is called 'junk'. The term is associated with foods originating in the fast-food chains of America rather than those coming from 'foody' France, home of the croque monsieur and foie gras, from Belgium, the country of moules et frites, or from Italy with its creamy pastas covered with cheese. For a century, generations of Britons ate fried fish and chips, liberally dosed with salt and vinegar, without becoming dangerously overweight. However, when the fish protein is replaced by the meat of a hamburger or by Kentucky Fried Chicken, it suddenly becomes a national disaster.

The present obsession with obesity has resulted in any food providing a high calorie content being labelled as 'junk'. It is obvious nonsense: cheese is good food, as are fish and chips and hamburgers. It is not the particular food that makes people fat, it is the amount of it that they eat. The whale is hugely fat – it is covered in fatty blubber – but it eats only plankton (which would no doubt qualify for the five-a-day portions of vegetables and fruit we are told we must eat). It is fat because it eats lots of plankton, not because plankton contains many calories. A person gorging themselves on fruit would become fat more quickly than one eating the occasional hamburger.

There is often confusion between so-called junk food and fast food. A pizza can provide an excellent meal even if it is likely to be a little heavy on fats, whereas a cherry tart that took hours to make is likely to contain more carbohydrate – even before the cream has been added to increase its fat content. Neither is junk, and both contribute food essential for the nourishment of the body.

So what is junk? I suppose the nearest one comes to a substance that is not nourishing is water. Nevertheless, a fluid intake of about two litres a day (some of it as water) is essential for survival. Fibre contributes so little towards our essential nutritional requirements that it could be considered a 'junk food', but of course it has a part to play in digestion. The lettuce and cucumber salad we are told we must eat every day to prevent us dying prematurely is made up of over 98 per cent water, while most of the rest is fibre and contributes little of nutritional value. We all know of children who have refused any salad or green vegetables and have grown up to be long-lived, healthy adults. Lettuce and cucumber would qualify for junk-food status but for the small amounts of water-soluble vitamins and antioxidants that they contain. Celery is said to require more energy in the eating than one gains from its consumption – that might qualify it for the label 'junk', but there is no evidence to suggest that it is in any way harmful.

It is clear that there is no such thing as junk food. It is a product of non-scientific pressure groups that, out of ignorance or prejudice, try to persuade us we are on the brink of a health catastrophe. The problem is not with the food we eat, but with the lifestyle of 'junk eaters'.

Chapter Eight

ORGANIC FOOD

BY STANLEY FELDMAN

The Myth: **Non-organic foods are covered in harmful pesticides.**

The Fact: **One of the pesticides deemed 'safe' by organic producers carries a warning that it is harmful to fish.**

Looking back to my childhood, it seems that every summer's day was sunny and filled with joy. I cannot remember it raining so hard that it spoiled a day out in the country. The food tasted better, the tomatoes were juicier, the strawberries sweeter and more succulent and the peas that came from the pods were so delicious that many were eaten raw before my mother could cook them. I realise, of course, that my memory is highly selective – there must have been rainy days, rotten tomatoes, sour strawberries and worm-infested peas, but somehow things today never seem quite as good as they were in our youth.

It is the same rose-tinted nostalgia that is used to promote 'organic food'. The cult of organic food is based on a belief that, while the sun may not always have shone in days gone by, the food was better and healthier before the advent of modern farming and horticulture, when the crops were liberally fertilised with manure from animal faeces or rotting vegetable waste in the form of compost.

The term organic food is in itself misleading. The separation into organic and inorganic was based on the belief that some substances contained a life-giving property: these were originally called 'organic'. In recent times it has come to mean chemicals containing molecules based on a carbon atom. So all food is organic (with the technical exception of water). There is no such thing as inorganic food. Whenever a pressure group resorts to a nonsense name in order to suggest that it has nature on its side, that it has the monopoly on what is good or that it is the only path that faithful followers of purity and truth can take, one should smell a rat.

The Soil Association, the high priests of this cult, believes that chemicals, whether organic or inorganic, are bad, a danger to the consumer and will possibly bring death to the planet. (In all fairness to them, it does permit the use of pesticides, providing they come from an approved list. Some have reassuringly innocent names such as 'soft soap', which turns out to be octodecanoic acid and carries a label warning that it is dangerous to fish.) Natural substances, by contrast, are apparently good. Yet all infections are caused by natural, organic bacteria; many organic substances produced in plants and berries, such as the belladonna of the deadly nightshade and the prussic acid in walnuts, are highly poisonous; the 'natural' copper sulphate that is recommended as a benign treatment for fungal infections is so toxic to marine life that treating boats with copper-based antifouling paints has been banned in many countries. If a fungicide is not used and the fungus therefore infects cereal crops, then the unsuspecting organic consumer may end up with gangrene of fingers and toes.

The main thrust of the argument used by adherents of this cult seems to be that organic fertiliser, by which it is implied that it is produced from animal excreta or rotting vegetable waste, is necessary in order to produce food that is both nutritious and safe. This supposition is difficult to support. It was reportedly Prince Albert who started the vogue for using natural, organic household waste to fertilise the kitchen garden at Osborne House on the Isle of Wight. Prince Albert died of typhoid fever, a disease caused by ingesting food contaminated with the faeces from a carrier who may not have exhibited symptoms of the disease. Manure is teeming with bacteria, many of which are pathogenic, and a few lethal. Compost rots because of the action of bacteria and, while these are in the main less harmful than those in manure, most sensible consumers would be reluctant to ingest them in the produce they purchase. The root systems of plants can only absorb nutrients that are in solution. They cannot take up particulate matter. Before the plant can use any fertiliser, organic faeces, rotting vegetable waste or chemical additive, it must first be broken down and rendered soluble in water. This necessitates organic matter being reduced to its basic chemical form. It is true that in organic fertiliser these are usually more complex chemicals, but they must be rendered into the same simple basic chemicals in the plant before they can be used to encourage its growth.

There is absolutely no rational reason why all the broken-down products of organic fertiliser should not be supplied in a basic chemical form rather than leaving it to the bacteria in the soil to produce them from compost. At the end of the day, the plant uses both chemical and organic fertiliser in the same way in the same chemical processes that are essential for its growth. The main difference is that chemical fertiliser is produced with a standardised value of its content, and does not contain the dangerous bacterial pathogens present in organic waste.

The other canon of organic law is the avoidance of known effective pesticides and the preference for naturally occurring compounds such as sulphur- or copper-based chemicals to control infestations. This again is illogical. It is based on the belief that the organophosphate pesticides are poisonous and naturally occurring chemicals are not, and ignores the fact that sulphur- and copper-based ones are also poisonous. Both organophosphate pesticides and naturally occurring chemicals can be poisonous, but it is all a matter of dose. To paraphrase the Swiss physician Paracelsus: nothing is without poison; it is the dose alone that makes it so.

The level of pesticides in our food is carefully monitored and kept below a very conservative safety level. The chemicals have a short half-life and have not been shown to accumulate in the body. Their level in food is way below that at which it is likely to cause symptoms, even in the most sensitive individual. Although pesticides in food have been blamed for a variety of ill-defined syndromes, extensive medical studies have failed to implicate them as the cause of any known clinical condition. There are no mysterious unknown diseases caused by the prolonged intake of small doses of these chemicals and, since they do not accumulate in the food chain or in the body, chronic toxicity is improbable.

The various conditions that have been attributed to these chemicals by the food faddists bear no relationship to any of the known effects of the pesticides. There have been sufficient cases of self-induced organophosphate poisoning to recognise the symptoms of poisoning (pesticides are a common form of suicide in Third World countries). It starts with excessive salivation and lachrymation and is invariably followed by painful gut cramps and an uncontrollable twitching of the muscles. Pesticides are not commonly associated with any allergic conditions. Virtually all the chemical pesticide residue that occurs in food is found on the outside of fruit and vegetables and is easily washed off.

When one looks at those parts of the world where pesticides are not freely available (usually because of cost) it is found that over a third of all the food produced is eaten by pests, whereas in the Western world, where pesticides are used, the loss is reduced by 41 per cent (figures from the WHO and the UN Environment Programme (1990)).

The inconsistent approach of the advocates of organic food becomes apparent when one considers organic eggs. These have to come from 'organic' chickens. To be an organic chicken, the bird has to eat 80 per cent organic food for six weeks. No effort is made to control the other 20 per cent, which may contain potential carcinogens or toxic material. At the end of that time, any eggs it lays will be organic and therefore much more expensive. Organic eggs and chickens should not be confused with free-range chickens that can eat whatever they like, are not kept in battery farms and probably enjoy a reasonably mixed diet.

There are many mysteries about what constitutes organic food. If a banana is squashed and its juice extracted to produce 'banana flavouring', it can be analysed and shown to be the chemical amyl acetate. However, if one produces amyl acetate by adding vinegar to amyl alcohol, it cannot be called 'organic'. It is the same chemical, it tastes the same and it smells the same, but it is not natural and it is therefore presumed to be bad. The same logic suggests that acetic acid is somehow different from the acid in vinegar, or citric acid from that of lemon juice extract.

A recent scare story has suggested that pre-packaged, cleaned lettuce is dangerous as it is washed in a solution containing chlorine. The initiates of this scare failed to point out that the amount of chlorine residue in the product is less than that found in most swimming-pool water and in some drinking water.

A walk around the organic shelves of a supermarket leaves one amazed at the gullibility of its patrons. There is no evidence that organic food is better for you than any other food. The Advertising Agency investigated the claim by organic farmers that their produce was 'healthier' and concluded that such a claim could not be justified. The produce is not particularly inviting in its appearance, and its taste is, for the most part, identical to that of the normal produce. Indeed, blind tasting has failed to reveal a consistent difference between organic and non-organic supermarket produce. This is hardly surprising, as taste is largely a result of the genetic make-up of the particular strain used, the time it has spent on the plant and the climatic conditions prevalent during its growth. Although most produce, be it organic or not, tastes better when freshly picked, the use of preservatives can prolong the freshness of some produce. Some preservatives are available for use in organic foods but they are seldom used in organic vegetables and fruits, which consequently have a short shelf life – as evidenced by wilting lettuces and bendy cucumbers.

Today, the zealots of the cult of organic food are making ever more irrational inroads into the way we live. They are promoting organic clothing and toiletries with the implied assurance that these are somehow less likely to cause allergies and skin disease. There is no scientific evidence to support this claim.

So why do people pay up to 50 per cent more for organic products? Is it a cynical confidence trick to exploit consumer ignorance? Is it the belief that, should little Johnny turn out to have allergies/asthma/autism or a brain tumour, this might have been prevented if he had been brought up on organic food and worn pyjamas made from organic cotton? Or is it simply a matter of choice? It is difficult to believe that the proponents of organic produce are part of an evil conspiracy to defraud the public, although they often use unworthy, unscientific scare tactics, conjuring up all sorts of disasters, to frighten the non-believers. Most just seem to be victims of their own propaganda, who yearn after bygone days when the sun shone all the time.

However, there is another side to the story. The food industry has to accept some of the blame. It has too often put cost before quality, marketed fruit picked before it has time to ripen and mature on the tree, and encouraged the production of food that looks good on the supermarket shelf rather than produce that tastes good when eaten. I believe that our memories of apples picked straight from the tree, tasting crisp and juicy, of strawberries that were sweet and succulent and peas that one could not resist eating raw have some factual basis. It is our desire to get back to the days of real, fresh, ripe fruit and vegetables that has encouraged the market for organic food.

Chapter Nine

SALT

BY SANDY MACNAIR

The Myth: **Eating less salt will reduce your blood pressure.**

The Fact: **A 30-year-old study shows that a low-salt diet may be linked to an increase in death from cardiovascular failure.**

It has long been received wisdom that too much salt in the diet is a cause of high blood pressure. In the days before we had effective drugs for treating high blood pressure, the salt-free 'rice and fruit' diet advocated by Kempner in 1944, although unpalatable, did help a few people lower the dangerously high blood pressure of malignant hypertension. It was less effective in the more common benign form of hypertension, and although it was suggested by Borst and Borst-de Gues in 1963 that this form of high blood pressure was due to an 'unwillingness' on the part of the kidneys to excrete salt, there is little to support their hypothesis.

The suggestion that salt intake affects the blood pressure of normal, healthy individuals has been made by various agencies, such as the WHO (1983). As evidence, they cite the fact that, in those societies with a high average salt intake, the mean blood pressure increases with age, whereas, in those whose salt consumption is low, such as the rainforest Indians of South America, there is no increase in blood pressure with age. This has led to governments in several countries making recommendations that the salt intake of the nation should be reduced. The evidence to support this edict is contentious.

A report entitled 'Dietary Reference Values for Food Energy and Nutrients for the United Kingdom' by the British government's Department of Health (1991) proposed that four grams of salt per day is sufficient for most people. In a further recommendation, in 'Nutritional Aspects of Cardiovascular Disease', the Department of Health (1994) recommended a reduction in daily salt intake from the current average of about nine grams to six grams.

SALT AND WATER: THE BACKGROUND

Over eons of time, water evaporated from the seas has fallen as rain, dissolving salt in the soil and carrying it down the rivers to the sea. As a result, salt is present in the oceans of the world at a concentration of some 35 grams per litre; thus 3.5 per cent of the total weight of the oceans of the world is salt. The Amazon alone discharges between 30 and 120 million litres of water per second. Not surprisingly, there is little salt left in the Amazon basin and the natives of the rainforest have had to adapt to the almost complete absence of salt in their diets. According to the Intersalt Study (1988), the Yanomamo tribesmen of Brazil each consume less than 15 milligrams of salt per day. In contrast, we in Britain have an average intake of about nine grams per day, or some 600 times as much.

THERMOREGULATION

Most of the energy produced in the animal body is dissipated as heat. This was uniquely important to *Homo sapiens* during his evolution. When man left the forest to live on the savannah, he added meat to his diet and had to be able to hunt for his food. This involved maintaining a high level of physical activity for a prolonged period. In order to be able to run for hours under a tropical sun without overheating, some means of producing heat loss was essential. This was achieved by sweating. It is why the evaporation of sweat is developed to such an unprecedented degree in man. No other mammal is known to sweat as much per unit of surface area. Man can produce an upper limit of about two litres of sweat per hour up to a maximum of 12 litres per day during prolonged exercise in the heat. There are about four million sweat glands dotted over the entire skin surface, and they can only function when there is an adequate concentration of salt in the blood.

Salt is essential to the process of sweating. Sodium pumps at the base of the sweat gland in our skin extract salt from the blood, the action of doing this drags water from the blood into the glands where it makes its way towards the surface of the skin. Some salt is reabsorbed along the sweat ducts in order to conserve sodium levels.

It is an oddity that man, who is the most dependent of all the mammals on evaporative water loss for thermoregulation, should have such a small capacity for consuming water. The legendary thirst of the camel allows it to drink up to 100 litres in 10 minutes; the smaller donkey can ingest 20 litres in three minutes; and even sheep can manage nine litres in 10 minutes. Man cannot drink much more than one litre in a 10-minute period. In these circumstances, we must assume that the earliest men used their superior intelligence to devise a means of carrying water on their hunting expeditions.

HOW MUCH SALT?

When one considers the importance of salt in both the evolution and the daily life of early *Homo sapiens*, it is ironic that an excess of salt in the diet is today supposed to be a threat to our health. Our ancestors when hunting, would be running for hours on end and would have produced up to two litres per hour with the maximum amount being about 12 litres a day. Being acclimatized to their environment (*see below*), their sweat would have contained about 1.25 grams per litre and they would need some 15 grams salt intake to replace the losses in sweat, let alone salt passed out in urine. It is likely that, as with modern man, salt intake, if freely available, tended to be well above the minimum requirement and the recommended intake for men working hard in very hot conditions today is 25 grams. So our ancestors must have consumed at least twice the average salt intake of present-day humans, and it would be reasonable to suppose that, having evolved with the ability to comfortably consume 25 grams per day, today's man is still able to handle a salt intake of nine grams without coming to much harm.

There are studies of the effects of such salt intake in modern man. One such study was by Jerome W Conn in 1944 on how the body acclimatises to a hot environment. Subjects were given over 30 grams of salt per day for several weeks, and he observed no apparent adverse effects. Conn discovered that nature's trick during acclimatization was to match the salt loss in the sweat produced to the customary salt intake of his test subjects. Unacclimatized subjects given an adequate supply of salt produce sweat that contains up to about six grams of salt per litre, and this decreases during acclimatisation.

Acclimatisation is achieved by increasing the rate of absorption of salt from sweat during its passage to the skin. Each of us tends to have a habitual salt intake which does not alter when we start to produce extra sweat on changing to hard work or a hot environment or both; the volume of sweat required as a daily average in the new circumstances depends on the average amount of heat to be dissipated. The process of acclimatization matches the unchanged habitual salt intake to the new level of water lost in sweat; salt intake and output come back into balance without the need to increase salt intake.

An important consequence of all this is that, in Britain's temperate maritime climate, few of us are acclimatized to hot weather. During a heatwave, we sweat and being unacclimatized we lose a great deal of salt in sweat. We recognise the water loss because we become thirsty and seek water to drink but the salt loss goes unnoticed and largely unreplaced. Thus, in a heatwave the elderly are very vulnerable to sodium depletion and reducing blood volume with consequent increases in blood viscosity and coagulability. Sudden deaths from arterial thrombosis (heart attack and strokes) among the older members of the population may increase dramatically in the few days following a heatwave. An adequate habitual salt intake clearly provides a defence against post-heatwave excess deaths.

Even those who are fully acclimatized need up to seven grams of salt each day. This figure coincides closely with the lowest salt intakes among those participants in the Intersalt Study who had free access to salt. It suggests that the average British intake of nine grams of salt per day is about right.

In 1978, Indiana University's Hypertension Research Centre (Murray *et al.* 1978) carried out studies on a group of eight volunteers who were given diets in which the daily salt content was increased every three days, from 0.6 grams initially, through 17 grams and 47 grams to a final level of 87 grams (about 10 times their normal intake). They were given plenty of water to drink, and they gained weight due to water retention. The mean blood pressure of the group rose from 110/66 mmHg to 130/85 mmHg on the highest intake – still within normal limits. Interestingly, one volunteer showed no change in his blood pressure over the whole range. Even with this enormous salt intake, they were troubled only by waking several times in the night with a full bladder!

SALT, WATER AND BLOOD PRESSURE

How can the intake of salt affect body water and blood pressure? An adult human has about 45 litres of body water, of which two-thirds is inside the cells – intracellular water – and the remaining third is extracellular, in the blood and around the cells. The concentration of sodium in the extracellular fluid is the dominant factor in determining the blood volume. This volume is regulated by various body systems and does not ordinarily fluctuate by more than 1 per cent. There are several feedback circuits which maintain the status quo.

The principal regulator of body water volume is the antidiuretic hormone (ADH) secreted by the pituitary gland when extracellular water volume is low. ADH conserves fluid by inhibiting the excretion of water by the kidneys. The hormone is released in response to a

rising sodium concentration in the blood. It also causes thirst, so
encouraging more water to be drunk. The principal guardian of the
sodium concentration in the extracellular fluid are the kidneys and
the nearby adrenal gland. They represent the centre of a very
complex and exquisitely tuned network that responds to changes in
blood volume, blood pressure and the extracellular concentration of
sodium, in order to keep each within its narrow normal range.
Professor Arthur Guyton and his colleagues at the University of
Mississippi carried out an exhaustive series of experiments on this
mechanism over many years and summarised their findings in a
review in 1989. They concluded that:

> Each person has a steady intake of salt, water and those other
> constituents that make up extracellular fluid. When the arterial
> pressure is normal, the kidney excretion of these constituents is
> exactly the correct amount to balance the intake of each of
> them. When the pressure is too great, there is more loss than
> gain, and the body fluid volume decreases; therefore, the
> pressure falls until the exact balance point is reached again; it is
> only at this balance point that the loss and gain are equal. At any
> pressure below the balance point, volume gain is greater than
> loss and the pressure will continue to rise until the exact balance
> level is again reached.

Guyton's studies show that, if a normal individual's salt intake is
suddenly raised by six or tenfold, then a kidney-based hormonal
system (the renin-angiotensin-aldosterone system, or RAAS) operates
to prevent even an extreme change in salt intake from having any
significant effect upon blood pressure. This complex system operates
slowly but with remarkable precision over the longer term.

However, the system is not able to respond to the effects brought
about by sudden changes. These situations require the much quicker,
self-regulating functions of the heart and blood vessels. The primary
function of the cardiovascular system is to circulate oxygenated

blood to the tissues. With the upright posture of the human, the brain is situated at the highest point in the body and is at the same time the most vulnerable to oxygen deprivation. If there were no means of keeping the blood supply to the brain constant, we would faint every time we stood up. The major blood vessels supplying the brain (the aorta and carotid arteries) are equipped with receptors which sense the pressure in the vessels. If the pressure falls below that required to keep the blood flowing to the brain, then signals from these receptors stimulate centres in the brain to increase sympathetic nervous drive, resulting in an immediate increase in rate and force of the heart, and contraction of blood vessels throughout the body. This produces a compensatory rise in blood pressure.

SALT–RESTRICTION TRIALS

It is fairly clear that the volume, pressure and ionic concentrations of the blood are very heavily defended by both local and systemic, nervous and hormonal feedback systems which compensate for wide variation in water and salt intake and for salt loss. However, none of these systems operates perfectly, as can be seen in results of a trial at Indiana University's Hypertension Research Center of the effects of salt restriction in normal healthy individuals (reported by Miller and colleagues in 1987). The dietary salt intake of 36 women and 46 men was reduced over a two-week run-in period. Their target was to get from the average American salt intake of nine grams per day to about half of that, and to maintain the new lower level for the three months of the study. The average salt intake was reduced from 9 to 3.9 grams per day during the trial and average blood pressure, which had been 107.3/71.7 mmHg at the beginning, was, after the 12 weeks on the salt-restricted diet, down by an average of an insignificant 1.7/1.9 mmHg. Very similar results were obtained in the most recent composite analyses of the numerous randomised trials of salt restriction.

Judy Miller and her colleagues published the changes in pressure for each individual. They demonstrated that, although 43 of the 82 subjects in the group showed little or no change, there were 25 whose pressure fell significantly (one by as much as 15 mmHg) and 14 who showed a significant rise in pressure (one as high as 17 mmHg). The responses presented a classic bell-shaped curve suggesting that, as with most biological feedback systems, there is a random variation in the efficiency and precision of the RAAS mechanism in any group of healthy people. The changes in blood pressure they noted did not match the changes in the loss of sodium in the urine. In a subsequent study involving 64 boys and 85 girls, very similar results were observed. In a 12-week period of salt restriction (down to less than 3.5 grams of salt per day), the blood pressure changes followed a similar bell-shaped curve with changes between +15 mmHg and –15 mmHg as in the adults, although in these children there was no change in the mean blood pressure.

SALT INTAKE AND HEART DISEASE

In a study in 1995 of the relationship between dietary salt intake and heart attacks among men with high blood pressure, Alderman *et al* followed up 2,937 subjects for an average of nearly four years. The incidence of heart attacks was recorded. They were lowest in the group with the highest salt intake. In another study in 1998, Alderman and his colleagues followed up the 11,348 Americans whose diet had been checked in the National Health and Nutrition Examination Survey of 1971–75. They found that the salt intake was inversely associated with deaths from all causes and especially with those deaths from cardiovascular disease: those with the lowest salt intakes showed the highest death rates. These studies do not prove that there is a hazard associated with a low-salt diet, but they give cause for concern in the absence of any studies showing the safety of salt restriction in terms of an improvement in cardiovascular death rates over the longer term.

One other cause for concern is reported in a study by Keatinge and his colleagues in 1986 into the marked rise in recorded deaths from heart attacks and strokes in a British heatwave in 1976. Maximum temperatures of 34.6°C were followed by peak mortalities from coronary and cerebral thrombosis one or two days later. They studied the effect on young, unacclimatized volunteers of exposing them to at 41°C for six hours during which time, despite ready access to water, they lost nearly two litres of sweat containing 12 grams of salt. In spite of water being freely available, the blood volume declined and the blood became thicker, a condition likely to promote arterial thrombosis in elderly people. Studies by the same group (Keatinge *et al*, 1984) showed that about half of the 60,000 excess deaths in winter are related to a thickening of the blood. Although the cases of deep-vein thrombosis and pulmonary embolism on long-haul flights are largely due to immobility, dehydration and a thickening of the blood are also clearly contributory. In all these instances, an adequate intake of salt along with fluid replacement will be protective.

CONCLUSION

The charge that is levelled is that we urbanised humans eat far more salt than is good for us and that it causes some, perhaps most of us, to develop high blood pressure as we grow older. This is intuitively improbable. Man, in his evolution from tree-dwelling vegetarian to the omnivorous hunter *Homo sapiens*, required an intake of salt above that of other primates. Left to his own devices, the average adult will take between six and 12 grams per day (Intersalt, 1988). There is no epidemiological evidence that salt intake is correlated with the prevalence of high blood pressure or that salt restriction will reduce blood pressure in young, normal individuals; indeed, it is clear that in a significant proportion of people (up to 20 per cent) the blood pressure may rise, sometimes alarmingly, if salt intake is reduced. For this reason it cannot be assumed that the reduction in salt intake by a population as a whole is either reasonable or safe. There is no evidence either of the efficacy or the safety of what appears to be the government policy of salt restriction in many developed countries, with the notable exception of Canada.

The champions of salt restriction across the population as a whole are, with a few exceptions, either nutritionists or epidemiologists who appear to understand neither the complexity nor the subtlety of the physiology involved in sodium and water homeostasis. Sodium is an essential nutrient and it is so important to the body that the unfortunate tribal peoples of the rainforests in such parts of the world as South America and Papua New Guinea have had to adapt to an environment in which there is virtually no natural presence of salt. This is evident from the high levels of the kidney hormone rennin in the blood, which stops them losing sodium in their urine. Although it is true that the blood pressure of these peoples does not rise as they get older, very few live to a ripe old age and their growth is stunted. On the other hand, the Japanese, whose average salt intake is among the highest in the world, are the longest-lived race in the world.

Because of the various feedback mechanisms which defend the blood pressure and maintain it within narrow limits, merely reducing the salt intake is almost certain to be without any significant effect on the blood pressure among the healthy, especially the young.

Salt restriction brings both the kidney and the sympathetic nervous control systems into play with powerful effects on the circulation. Due to an overshoot in this mechanism, many healthy individuals show a significant increase in blood pressure when salt is restricted. Without adequate randomised trials to establish its long-term safety, and in particular to show reduced cardiovascular mortality, the imposition of a low-salt diet by government dictat appears foolhardy and without sound scientific basis.

Chapter Ten

WATER

BY STANLEY FELDMAN

The Myth: **We should make an effort to drink two litres of water every day.**

The Fact: **Most of that two litres is already supplied in the food we eat.**

It seems that a bottle of water has become a fashion accessory, with young people binge drinking its contents at every occasion. Are we in the midst of yet another 'epidemic', one that dehydrates us to such an extent that we need constantly to top up our body's water level?

It is difficult to discover how this unlikely fashion started. The fluid needs of the body have been known for over 50 years, and we have managed to survive without swigging water at every opportunity. Perhaps the fashion can be traced back to the WHO's quite reasonable suggestion that about two litres a day of clean water is required, in addition to other nutritional needs, for all adults. There is evidence that the bottled-water industry has taken this as the basis of a sales pitch. In a recent BBC broadcast (*You and Yours*, December 2004) their representative insisted that water *meant* water, and out of preference it should be bottled water. Other fluids would not do, because they were not the pure 'clean water' referred to by the WHO.

WATER BALANCE

Let's look at the reason behind our need for water. Life began in the oceans where water was plentiful. Only millions of years later, when the salt content of the seas increased to toxic levels, did a desalination mechanism become necessary in order to prevent a build-up of salt in the body. The kidneys carried out this function. When life emerged from the seas on to land, access to water became difficult and conservation of fluid became the priority for the kidney. As land-based life developed its ability to forage for food, a need to rid the body of excessive quantities of other salts and chemicals contained in this new diet, became necessary. Although the kidney became the principal organ for removing these unwanted substances from the body, it still retained the ability to conserve water by concentrating the urine. As the kidney can only excrete water-soluble chemicals, it needs a supply of water to fulfil this function. The amount of water required will depend on the amount of waste substances produced as a result of metabolism and the efficiency of the kidney at concentrating the urine.

Man is particularly vulnerable to a shortage of water: it is not only essential so that the chemicals that are the end product of metabolism can be excreted in the urine, it is also a crucial part of our heat-loss mechanism. Out of every 100 calories we burn in our bodies at rest, about 80 calories end up as heat. In order to cope with this inevitable heat production, man has evolved into a very sweaty organism – it is principally by the evaporation of sweat that we lose heat. The dangers associated with an inability to sweat have been known since ancient times, when god figures often died after they were covered from head to toe in gold paint for ceremonial purposes. More recently it was found that patients encased in whole body plasters often developed dangerously high temperatures. Sweating is so efficient that a man can exist in a room hot enough to cook a steak providing the atmosphere is dry; however, if the humidity is high and sweat cannot evaporate, he will die. Even at a room temperature of 20°C we lose heat by sweating – one does not have to be pouring with sweat to lose significant amounts of water. It is estimated that in temperate climates the average adult loses about 500 millilitres of water as sweat without even being aware of the loss. The loss of water will be higher if he or she does hard physical work, or if the ambient temperature is raised.

We also lose water during breathing. We breathe relatively dry air into our lungs, and exhale fully saturated moist air. One only has to breathe out on to a cold mirror to demonstrate the amount of water contained in our breath. The more rapidly and deeply we breathe, the more the water is lost in this way. In normal circumstances we lose about 500 millilitres of water every 24 hours by this means.

Most of our water loss, however, is from the kidneys. The amount is variable as it depends upon the food we eat and the efficiency of the kidneys at concentrating urine. An average person on a mixed diet loses between 800 millilitres and one litre of fluid by this means.

A litre from the kidneys, half a litre through the breath and half a litre through sweating: we can now see where the fluid requirement of two litres a day comes from. It is neither a minimum nor a maximum figure as the amount needed varies with lifestyle, ambient temperature and the amount of physical work done.

FLUID INTAKE

With a normal mixed diet we take in about one litre of fluid as an inevitable consequence of the food we eat. A cucumber is 98 per cent water; fruit, seafood and fish are about 80–90 per cent water, and even meat contains about 20–30 per cent water – one only has to leave a piece of fresh meat out of the refrigerator for a few hours to see how much fluid oozes out. Some meats have added water injected into them: ham, bacon, turkey and chicken often have up to 30 per cent of their weight added as water. Only those on a very low-roughage, high-protein diet, or those on a starvation slimming diet, fail to take in at least one litre of fluid with their food. If in addition one drinks a bowl of soup and two cups of tea or coffee, or a glass of beer a day, one will have fulfilled the body's fluid requirement.

Is there any harm in drinking extra water? Not really, except that it means extra trips to the toilet, and there are a few – usually elderly – people in whom the brain's control system that normally adjusts our thirst to our fluid needs is not robust and who may suffer a water overload.

Is there any time we need more than two litres of fluid a day? If the ambient temperature is high, the loss through sweating is increased even though one may not be aware of it; if the body temperature is raised, for example during a fever, extra water and salt is essential; if the rate of metabolism is increased during exercise, heat is produced and extra water may be necessary to replace that lost in sweating; and if breathing is increased, for example to meet the needs of physical work or as part of the adaptation to a high altitude, then there will be additional water loss and the need for an increased intake.

But, provided one is living a normal lifestyle and eating a sensible mixed diet, there is no need to carry around a bottle of water. One can be reassured that it is very unusual for fit people in temperate climates to suffer from dehydration. We have an exquisitely sensitive mechanism that tells us when we need to drink more fluid: it is called thirst.

Chapter Eleven

ALCOHOL

BY VINCENT MARKS

The Myth: **Alcohol is a dangerous health risk.**

The Fact: **Moderate alcohol intake increases longevity.**

Alcohol is both a food and a drug of addiction; it is the problems associated with the latter that attracts media attention. This essay will address both of its properties.

Man's use of alcohol dates back to pre-history. Beer was brewed from cereals in Egypt as long ago as 5000 BC. Distillation was used to make what we now call spirits in China 3,000 years ago, although it did not reach Europe until around the fifteenth century. Today, alcohol is used in every country in the world, even where it is forbidden by law on religious grounds.

Customs and Excise records relating to alcohol go back to 1680, and show just how much it contributed to the diet at that time. Average daily consumption in 1700, the peak year, was sufficient to provide about 50 grams (six units) per head for the total population (including men, women and children). It was taken almost entirely in the form of beer and was probably the only drink free from bacterial contamination available to town dwellers. Alcoholic drinks must have contributed 20 per cent or more of the daily calorie intake, compared with about 6 per cent today. Even this relatively small amount is significant and should be taken into account in any calculation of energy intake. Beer brewed in former times contained a substantial proportion of the daily vitamin and mineral requirements, although this is not the case nowadays – few beers contain more than trace amounts of these substances; spirits contain none at all, and are the original source of the 'empty-calories' concept.

Britain still consumes far less alcohol than many other countries. The current record is held by the Irish. The French, who were the world leaders in alcohol consumption, and took it mainly in the form of wine, have reduced their consumption by 40 per cent in the past 30 years; our consumption, still made up mainly of beer, has gone up by an equivalent amount. Alcohol intake reached its nadir in Britain between 1945 and 1950, when it was around one half of its present level. Since then it has risen slowly but inexorably. This has largely been due to an increased consumption of wine, which until recent times was considered a luxury, enjoyed by the rich.

Alcohol intake varies from one part of the country to another, and between different communities. Scotland has a higher alcohol intake per head than south-east England, but it also has a higher proportion of teetotallers. This may be due to the particular type of alcohol abuse prevalent among the Scots and other northern Europeans that can be described as 'drinking to get drunk', leading to signing of a pledge not to do so by those who have seen or experienced the aftermath. In contrast, the people of the Mediterranean take their alcohol, mainly in the form of wine, with their meals. This gives rise to a very different type of alcohol abuse.

THE PROS AND CONS OF ALCOHOL

Unlike in times gone by when beer and spirits were the only germ-free drinks available, alcohol owes its present popularity to its pharmacological effect. It causes euphoria and reduces inhibitions.

It is possible to draw up a balance sheet pitting the good effects of alcohol against the unfavourable ones. It is the unfavourable effects that dominate the attention given to alcohol in the media. It is this, together with their personal experience, upbringing and genetic propensity, that formulates people's attitude to alcohol. It is strange that, whereas two of the three great monotheistic religions use alcohol in their rituals, the third forbids any contact with it.

Alcohol abuse is one of the main causes, if not *the* main cause, of antisocial behaviour. This can take the form of public drunkenness, irresponsible behaviour, especially by members of a crowd, and violence towards oneself as well as others. Alcohol impairs work performance even when taken in modest amounts. Anyone who has counted the number of errors they make while using a computer after drinking even a very small amount of alcohol with their lunch will have personal experience of this. The banning of alcohol on university campuses and other work places at lunchtime has much to be said for it – alcohol and work just do not go together.

Currently, over 90 per cent of men and 85 per cent of women in Britain drink alcohol at least occasionally, and 6 per cent and 2 per cent respectively drink the equivalent of more than a bottle of wine a day. In a survey conducted in 1997, 12 per cent of young men and 5 per cent of young women between the ages of 16 and 24 admitted being drunk once a week during the previous three months. The percentage is probably higher today. Three-quarters of all stabbings and two-thirds of all murders in Britain are committed under the influence of alcohol, as are half of all street crimes and a third of sexual offences. Chronic alcohol abuse is the commonest cause of domestic violence and is responsible for many family break-ups.

Fifteen per cent of road-traffic deaths are associated with excessive alcohol use, either by drivers of cars and motorcycles, or by pedestrians. This is less than it was before the campaign against drink-driving got under way some 30 years ago, but it is still too high. Many of the offenders are chronic alcoholics whose compulsion to drink is so great that they either do not recognise their impairment or are indifferent to it. Many are otherwise decent, ordinarily law-abiding people who do not appreciate that one does not have to be drunk for one's judgement to be impaired. The legal limit in the UK for alcohol in the blood is a pragmatic compromise. It is 40 per cent higher than that recommended for safety.

Few people realise how much alcohol they can drink over a given time and still remain within our liberal drink-driving restrictions. The unit system has gone some way towards helping us understand the effect of alcohol intake on the level of alcohol in the blood. One unit in the UK is about 10 millilitres or eight grams of pure alcohol and is the amount contained in a single 25-millilitre measure of spirits. It is substantially less than the amount of alcohol contained in half a pint of good-quality beer or quarter of a pint of strong cider. An average 120-millilitre glass of wine contains nearly one and a half units of alcohol, and the 250-millilitre glasses now served in some pubs provide three units. Four units of alcohol taken on an empty stomach can bring a man weighing 70 kilograms dangerously near the UK limit for driving, and well above it in countries with lower limits.

A typical person disposes of alcohol, by destroying it in their liver, at a rate of around eight grams – or one unit – an hour. The exact rate varies and is largely determined by one's genes. Nothing one can do will increase it, although some drugs decrease it. Alcohol drunk hours earlier may still be present in the body long after it might be supposed to have disappeared, especially in people who metabolise it slowly. This is why some drivers, after a moderate-to-heavy drinking session the night before, may be above the legal limit the morning after. They won't feel drunk, but they will be impaired.

However, the adage 'don't drink and drive' may be unduly restrictive. The effect of alcohol on the mind depends upon the amount drunk and whether it is taken with food. Assuming that no alcohol had been taken in the previous 12 hours, it is possible for an average man to have a 'starter', such as a sherry, and then drink half a bottle of wine (three units) at the rate of one unit per hour with a meal and remain within the legal limits. These amounts are unsafe, however, when drunk on an empty stomach, and need to be reduced by a third for women weighing less than 70 kilograms. And just because a driver is legally 'safe', he is not necessarily a safe driver, as his reaction time at alcohol levels well below the legal limit will be slowed, especially if he is a naïve drinker.

It is not only the damage that alcohol does to society through its effect upon behaviour, but also its effects upon health that make it a concern. The causal links between chronic excessive alcohol consumption and cirrhotic liver disease is so well established that the prevalence of cirrhosis in a society has been used as a marker for alcoholism. Other organs that can be affected by alcohol are the pancreas, bones, blood, the various endocrine glands and of course the nervous system where, in its most malignant form, it produces permanent and irreversible damage. There is some weak epidemiological evidence linking alcohol use to various types of cancer, mostly of the mouth and upper alimentary tract, but an increased incidence at more distant sites, apart from the liver, is difficult to reconcile with the much-promoted anti-cancer effect of the antioxidants in many alcoholic drinks.

With such a weight of evidence against alcohol, is there anything to be said in its favour? Should it not be banned as a dangerous drug of addiction that causes far more ill health and deaths than cannabis, cocaine and heroin combined?

Not only was the impracticability of this demonstrated by the failure of prohibition in America; the desirability of doing so is far from established. To ban the use of alcohol would deny us access to what is possibly a health-promoting, therapeutic agent. Leaving aside the fact that the alcohol industry is one of the largest employers of labour in the country and makes an enormous contribution to the economy as well as to our export and internal revenues, there is very good evidence that, used properly, alcohol increases longevity and prevents some of our commonest diseases, as well as providing the lubrication of social intercourse.

Life assurance companies have known for generations that moderate alcohol use is associated with longevity. It is only in the past 30 years or so that this has been established as being due to its effect on reducing deaths from coronary heart disease. It probably also reduces the incidence of type-2 diabetes, an increasingly important cause of chronic illness, invalidity and death.

The evidence for the beneficial effects of alcohol upon coronary heart disease comes from an ever-growing list of epidemiological studies from all over the developed world that is consistent with age-old evidence from autopsies carried out on chronic alcoholics. These autopsies found that, whatever else may have ailed them, the coronary arteries of alcoholics were generally unusually free from disease. The effect is more or less specific to the coronary arteries and aorta. How alcohol exerts its beneficial effects, and whether it is the alcohol itself or some substances associated with it in alcoholic beverages, is not known.

One of the strongest cases that can be made for the beneficial effects of alcohol is its action in raising the concentration of the high-density lipoproteins (HDL) in the blood. HDLs carry what is often referred to as 'good' cholesterol, and there is reliable evidence that this cholesterol is linked to a reduced risk of coronary artery disease. Although far from proven, there is a suggestion that alcohol from wine is more beneficial than that from beer or spirits, although all sources seem to confer some benefit. The most ardent advocates of the benefits of wine-drinking attribute it mainly to the antioxidants, more of which are to be found in red than in white wine. Indeed, wine is an important constituent of the so-called Mediterranean diet, which dietary experts have declared to be healthy.

Against these very positive effects of alcohol must be weighed the fact that it is one of the commonest preventable causes of high blood pressure, and it contributes to strokes.

The evidence regarding what constitutes an optimum alcohol intake is reasonably clear. For men it is about two to four units a day, for women one to three. The level at which the health benefits are outweighed by the penalties are less clear. Few studies have tackled this problem, but one, which has involved a 15-year follow-up of

36,000 healthy men in Nancy, France, suggested that an alcohol intake of up to 30 grams was associated with a substantially longer life expectancy; up to 60 grams of alcohol a day, or twice the optimum, produced the same life expectancy as lifelong teetotalism. It would seem that drinking two to three glasses of wine (three to four units) a day increases life expectancy but drinking over five glasses (six to seven units) reduces it.

What defines alcoholism? There is no universally acceptable definition since alcohol can produce problems in so many different ways. It is probably better just to speak of alcohol abuse. I believe that anyone who incurs a personal health penalty, or produces social disruption, by drinking alcohol is abusing it. The level of alcohol at which this occurs varies from one individual to another and on the circumstances in which it is taken. Regular consumers of more than one bottle of wine a day – or six alcohol units taken in any form – must be putting themselves at an unacceptable risk whereas those drinking just half that amount can be considered prudent and health-conscious.

Accepting that the evidence linking alcohol consumption in moderate amounts (from as few as seven units a week to as many as 28 and possibly 40 units a week for a man) with health benefits is convincing, are there any people who ought not to drink at all? The answer is undoubtedly yes. Those with a strong family history of alcoholism would be better off never starting to drink rather than running the risk of being unable to stop. Those who have already had difficulties with alcohol are better off becoming completely abstinent rather than trying to moderate their drinking which most find impossible. Others who should not drink are patients receiving prescription drugs that interact with alcohol. These are too numerous to mention by name, but the common blanket prohibition of alcohol to patients prescribed antibiotics is unjustified except in special circumstances.

Pregnant women – or to be more precise their foetuses – are especially at risk from a devastating condition known as the foetal alcohol syndrome and the more common but infrequently diagnosed condition of foetal alcohol effects, a common cause of preventable mental handicap. Quantities of alcohol that present no danger to the non-pregnant woman can do so to a foetus. The occasional binge drinker is as much at risk as the chronic alcoholic. No one knows at what stage of a pregnancy the foetus is most vulnerable or at what level of alcohol intake it becomes a problem, so to cover their own backs some doctors advise total abstinence from alcohol during pregnancy. This advice, which is almost certainly unjustified on the evidence, imposes an unnecessary burden of guilt on women who may have drunk the occasional glass of wine before they had been warned of the risks or known they were pregnant.

Telling the truth about the advantages as well as the disadvantages of alcohol as a constituent of our diet and letting people make their own judgements is, I believe, a better option than that advocated by the World Health Organisation who take the view that the health advantages of alcohol relative to its disadvantages have not been unequivocally established. This may be true from the point of view of society as a whole, but to the vast majority of people who use alcohol moderately and intelligently it produces an undeserved sense of guilt. The fact is that alcohol is here to stay, and we must learn how to use it wisely.

Chapter Twelve

SUGAR

BY VINCENT MARKS

The Myth: Sugar causes coronary heart disease, diabetes, hypertension, gout, tooth decay and obesity.

The Fact: It only really contributes to tooth decay and its adverse effects can be offset by the addition of fluoride to drinking water and toothpaste.

Sugar has had a bad press: the nutritionist Professor John Yudkin has described it as 'pure, white and deadly'. A whole episode of the BBC's flagship current-affairs programme *Panorama* on 10 October 2004 was devoted to the supposed iniquities of the sugar industry. The reason for this media interest is that we know we do not need sugar in our diet in order to survive – we can live perfectly good, healthy lives without it. Nevertheless, we like it. The question is, does it do us any harm?

Sugar means different things to different people. To a doctor or nurse, sugar in a medical context is synonymous with glucose, because it is the only simple sugar found in body fluids such as blood and urine in amounts that are easily measured. It is the form in which the sugar we eat is used by the body. To a chemist, sugar is an alternative name for one type of carbohydrate. These are carbon-containing compounds in which hydrogen and oxygen occur in the same ratio as in water. They are usually sweet to the taste. To the cook, sugar is synonymous with sucrose, a substance containing equal amounts of glucose and fructose bound to one another chemically and comes either from sugar cane or sugar beet. Both produce sugar that is indistinguishable without the help of sophisticated isotopic analysis.

However, to those in the food industry not all sugars are sucrose. To them the term 'sugar' includes both sucrose and invert sugar. Invert sugar is made from sucrose by splitting it chemically into an equal mixture of fructose and glucose. More recently, something resembling invert sugar has been made from hydrolysed starch. It contains more fructose than glucose and is cheaper than ordinary sugar. It is widely used in the soft-drinks industry in the USA, and to some extent in Europe.

All the sugar we buy in the shops is sucrose. In its unrefined state it is inedible and brown. So-called 'natural brown sugar' is partially purified sugar, which still contains some plant colourants. It is sold at a premium to people who believe it is better for them than white sugar. It's not the same as conventional brown (table) sugar, which is ordinary refined white sugar, stained brown.

There is absolutely no reason why sucrose, taken as sugar, should figure in our diet at all. Unlike proteins, fats, vitamins, minerals and water, it is not an essential constituent of our diet, but its presence in all fruit and most commercially prepared foods makes it extremely difficult to avoid. The transformation of sugar from an expensive luxury in the seventeenth century to a substance providing some 10 per cent or more of our average daily energy intake is due principally to its sweetness. It is seldom used primarily as a source of calories as it is always more expensive than starchy or fatty foods. Despite the current fashion for low-carbohydrate diets, some carbohydrate is probably necessary. Starch, the most abundant carbohydrate in all but the most bizarre diets, can be converted by the body into all the various forms of sugar required by the body as part of its structure as well as for energy.

Sweetness is a primary taste. Mother's milk contains lactose, a sugar with about one half of the sweetness of sucrose, and many synthetic milk preparations contain sucrose – it is added to make cow's milk, which has only half the lactose content of human milk, more palatable. It is this ability to make foods and medicines palatable that has led to sugar's current widespread use and production throughout the world.

No one would come to physical harm if they never ate another gram of sugar. Indeed, there is a rare disease, more common in western France and Switzerland than in Britain, that can only be treated effectively by completely excluding sugar from the diet. This necessitates avoiding fruits and many vegetables as well as foods containing refined sugar. This disease – hereditary fructose intolerance – provides good evidence for the non-essential nature of dietary sucrose and fructose: sufferers can lead healthy lives providing they avoid fructose, and because they cannot eat sugar they usually have very healthy teeth. This demonstrates the importance of sucrose in producing dental decay – the one genuine common ailment that can be laid at its door.

Sugar was considered a highly desirable dietary item until comparatively recently. The idea that it might not be all it was cracked up to be, and that it could be a cause of bad rather than good health, appears to have gained ground during the 1950s. It was promoted by a British naval officer, Surgeon Captain Cleave, who in 1957 coined the name 'saccharine disease' to describe a number of seemingly unrelated chronic illnesses that he attributed to the large amounts of highly refined carbohydrates in the diet. These included not only sugar but also white flour and polished rice, all of which had had much of their health-promoting factors removed, leaving behind just empty calories. Professor John Yudkin, one of the most distinguished academic nutritionists in Britain at the time, working independently of Cleave, also came down heavily on the detrimental effects of sugar in his book *Pure, White and Deadly*. He exonerated dietary starches because they only produce glucose following digestion in the gut. He believed that it was largely the fructose component of table sugar that was harmful.

Cleave and Yudkin both relied heavily on epidemiological evidence linking increased sugar use with a rising incidence of coronary heart disease, diabetes, hypertension, gout, tooth decay and of course obesity. Cleave went further and included peptic ulceration, varicose veins and diverticulitis of the colon among the various manifestations of the saccharine disease that he blamed in part upon the loss of dietary fibre during the refining process.

The rise in life expectancy in the past 50 years has been associated with an increase in the prevalence of chronic diseases. The possible link between diet and disease has led to attempts by governments on both sides of the Atlantic to find out if changes to our diet might make us healthier. In the USA, a committee chaired by George McGovern published its 'Dietary Goals for the United States' in 1977. The main thrust of the report was that Americans should reduce their fat, cholesterol and meat intake and increase their carbohydrate consumption to a level such that it would provide 55–60 per cent of their total energy (calorie) intake. These changes were to be achieved by increasing the consumption of fruits, vegetables and whole grains, while reducing the intake of refined sugar to 15 per cent of total energy intake (this was amended in the second edition, published later in the year, to 10 per cent).

This figure was not based on any hard scientific evidence. Though the target may have been achievable, it was not reached. Indeed, there is no evidence that it would have done most of those reaching the target much good. It might possibly have reduced their incidence of tooth decay and, if combined with other dietary restrictions, lessened the risk of obesity. Similar advice was offered by NACNE (National Advisory Committee on Nutrition Education) – an ad hoc British committee whose final report was never issued officially. (It was claimed that it was never officially endorsed, due to a dirty-tricks campaign by the food industry.)

In the 1980s, behavioural disorders in children were added to the list of diseases that Cleave and Yudkin had ascribed to sugar. As a result of this crescendo of accusations about the role of sugar in disease, the Centre for Food Safety and Applied Nutrition commissioned the most thorough evaluation of the health aspects of sugars and sweeteners ever undertaken. The Food and Drug Administration (FDA) Sugars Task Force took into account that in America, but not in Europe, only half of the sugar consumed per head of the population was sucrose; the rest was largely high-fructose corn syrup (HFCS), whose production in Europe was held back to protect the sugar beet industry. If fructose was the real culprit, these studies should have revealed it. The task force found that there was absolutely no evidence that sugar, including those sugars with a high fructose content, caused any of the long list of diseases laid at its door, including diabetes and behavioural disorders in children. The only exception was tooth decay (this problem has been partly overcome in the UK by the addition of fluoride to drinking water and toothpaste). Only in the case of hereditary fructose intolerance and a few other equally rare genetic disorders can sugar be considered a specific health risk.

This is not the impression given by most health writers, who do themselves and their readers a disservice by extrapolating from animal experiments, in which huge amounts of sugars are added to animals' diets, to human beings eating a normal diet. There probably are some people, especially but not exclusively children, who drink inordinately large amounts of sugary drinks or eat too many sweets. People often do not realise how much sugar they consume in various products, especially in fruits and fruit juices. One grossly obese patient told me that she drank four litres of pure fruit juice a day. What she did not realise was that this contained 400 grams of sugar providing 1,600 calories, even though no sugar or syrup had been added. While it is true that sugar in fruit is associated with trace elements, vitamins and dietary fibre, whereas sugar from a packet or in prepared foods is not, the sugar in both is exactly the same.

The way in which sugar is eaten does, however, have an effect upon some functions of the body. Taken in large amounts on an empty stomach, sugar, especially glucose, can cause such a sudden rise in the blood-sugar level that it produces an excessive corrective response producing a fall to a level that may temporarily interfere with brain function. This condition, referred to as 'reactive hypoglycaemia', is easy to produce in the laboratory, but rare in real life. It became a fashionable condition in the 1970s – when a diagnosis of hypoglycaemia was in vogue, which was more socially acceptable than the generally more realistic ones of neurosis, chronic alcoholism or anxiety states. Hypoglycaemia provided a bonanza for health writers who could lay at sugar's door yet another supposed evil. They even went so far as to describe sugar as a poison or toxin that ruined the lives of millions of unsuspecting victims. They claimed, without scientific evidence, that removing sugar from the diet cured these conditions. Today a diagnosis of hypoglycaemia is largely confined to rare cases of disease affecting one or more of the bodily organs and produces a low concentration of glucose in the blood.

There is no doubt that sugar makes food palatable and in this sense contributes to obesity, which is an important cause of diabetes and heart disease. It is sensible to try to reduce the intake of sugar in children especially in carbonated soft drinks as large amounts make them fat and cause dental decay. Adults should make their own choice whether to drink water, fruit juice or unsweetened drinks, provided that they make their choice knowingly and not on the basis of spurious benefits suggested by an advertisement. There is no specific health reason why access to sugary products should be limited, and people preferring them should not be made to feel guilty by those who improperly condemn sugar as a noxious substance. After all, as Mary Poppins reminds us, a spoonful of sugar helps the medicine go down!

Chapter Thirteen

PESTICIDES IN FOOD

BY LAKSHMAN KARALLIEDDE

'A person injured by a burning firewood panics on seeing
the harmless white light of a firefly.'

AN OLD SRI LANKAN SAYING

The Myth: Our food is doused in harmful pesticides.

The Fact: Pesticide residues are not allowed to exceed one-hundredth of the amount
that causes even a slight reaction in the most sensitive species.

The public is justifiably concerned by reports of the horrendous
consequences of food contaminated with pesticides. What are the
facts and how far are these horror stories justified?

Pesticides have been manufactured with the intent of destroying
life – that of the pests, insects, weeds and fungi that destroy crops and
reduce their yield. These infestations are a major factor contributing
to global malnutrition. Pesticides were initially introduced to destroy
those insects that are the vectors of diseases such as malaria,
bilharzia, trachoma and fly-borne gastroenteritis. Malaria alone
causes huge global misery: each year it causes as many as 3,000,000
deaths and about 5,000,000,000 episodes of clinical illness
necessitating anti-malarial therapy with children in Africa suffering

between four and five episodes of febrile illness, assumed to be malaria, every year. Fly-borne gastroenteritis is the biggest single killer of children in Africa.

Pesticides are dangerous. Ill health and deaths have been caused by the oral intake of large quantities of insecticides by people trying to commit suicide. Although common in Asia and South America, such incidents are rare in developed countries where pharmaceutical agents and toxic household products are more likely to be used by those attempting suicide. Just as the careless use of a car may lead to death and injury (globally, 25 per cent of all 'injuries' are road-traffic related), the misuse of pesticides will cause ill health. In contrast to cars, pesticides are used mainly by those with a poor educational and scientific background. Ignorance and misunderstanding leads to misuse. In many parts of the world no licensing is required and no training offered to those responsible for spraying crops with pesticides. It is often impoverished, illiterate farmers living in developing countries, some on the verge of starvation, who carry out the spraying of pesticides. They often live in single-room dwellings where they cook, eat and store the pesticide alongside their food. Their primary aim is to generate sufficient income from their produce for the survival of their families. The vast majority of them know nothing about the toxicity of the pesticides they use, and apply these dangerous chemicals, frequently in uncontrolled mixtures, in amounts that often exceed those recommended. They cannot afford to buy any of the necessary protective gear or to obtain modern spraying equipment. There is a sense of desperation which forces them to take risks and work much longer hours than are acceptable in developed countries. They frequently spray pesticides all day, with a total disregard to weather conditions and wind direction.

Under these circumstances it is not surprising that there are cases of ill health among those using pesticides. There have also been reports of poisoning that has occurred following the accidental contamination of food. Virtually all these instances of contamination have taken place in poverty-ridden communities where facilities for the safe, separate storage of pesticides are beyond the reach of the populace.

Accidental contamination of this kind in Asia and South America is very different from the problem of pesticide residues in the food eaten in developed countries. The former implies some form of pollution, involving much larger amounts of pesticides than those found as 'residues'. The presence of a 'residue' implies a much less harmful situation, either because of the circumstance in which it occurs or the amount involved. Although there have been reports of food contaminated with naturally occurring toxins from plants and bacteria, and from chemical contamination, causing ill health and even death in developed countries, there are no reports of any such effect ever being caused by the residues of pesticides. The scenarios of ill health and danger due to pesticides are entirely a result of unusual, unacceptable and unfortunate practices that are rife in developing countries. They are not encountered in developed countries like the UK where regulatory and monitoring process are active, aggressive and advanced.

HOW MUCH PESTICIDE?

The use of pesticides on edible crops and in horticulture is controlled in the European Union by Directive 91/414.

In technologically advanced countries such as the UK, pesticide residues are constantly monitored, using the most advanced equipment available to ensure that the public are provided with a consistent supply of high-quality clean food, free of unwanted chemicals. Various factors are taken into consideration, such as the acceptable daily intake (ADI). This is the amount of a pesticide which can be consumed safely every single day of one's life. To arrive at this there are studies of the absorption rate of the chemical, its distribution and the way in which it is metabolised and excreted. This is then set against all the known data for its toxicity. The actual dose accepted is calculated from information gathered from the most sensitive endpoint in the most sensitive species. The level of safety found in these tests is then usually reduced a hundredfold to give the acceptable maximum level, the ADI, in food. This hundredfold reduction in the acceptable toxicity comprises a factor of 10 for potential interspecies extrapolation and a further 10 for interspecies variability. Where the pesticide has appreciable acute toxicity (the sort of chemical only used in exceptional cases as a single dose) a second reference dose is given. This is the acute reference dose (ARfD) and is the amount of a pesticide which, on the basis of current knowledge, can be consumed with complete safety at a single meal or in a single dose. The calculations are done separately for toddlers and adults.

The maximum residue level of pesticide, the MRL, is derived from field trials data. The pesticide is used at the maximum recommended rate, and the crop is analysed for residues. The MRL is then calcuated from the residues. The MRL must also be consistent with safety for the consumer. From dietary surveys, there are data on food intake for the UK population and for sub-populations such as toddlers. The intake figures for an extreme consumer (usually the 95 percentile) are multiplied by the MRL and the product should be less than the ADI and, for an acute risk assessment, the ArfD. In addition, the MRL values are based on an overgenerous allowance of food consumption per day. Already low residue levels of pesticides are, in practice, even lower, because in order to reach the agreed limit you would have to consume an indecent amount of food. Occasional instances where the MRL has been exceeded have been seized upon in the media as evidence of a dangerous failure of the system. They interpret the MRL as a safety limit. It is not: it is derived from trials data and, in the case of most crop/pesticide combinations, the MRLs can be comfortably exceeded, without the ADI or ArfD being exceeded. Exceeding the MRL indicates a failure to use pesticides correctly, but as an isolated incident it should not give rise to any concern to the consumer.

The toxic effects of organophosphorus insecticides are well documented. Scaremongers have speculated that long exposure to low doses may be responsible for virtually all of the medical problems suffered by humanity (as well as the early demise of thousands of animal, bird and plant species). They have fostered fears of carcinogenicity and birth defects in spite of an absence of any toxicology data to substantiate their claims. The fact that the only scientific report that relates low-dose exposures (as opposed to doses taken orally with suicidal intent) to any medical problem has followed the occupational use of pesticides by those involved in preparing the solutions used for sheep dips seems to have passed them by. There is no evidence to suggest that long-term exposure to the minuscule amounts of pesticides on some produce is likely to cause any ill effects. There have never been any reports of any effects on health due to pesticide residues on food, even when it exceeded the MRL.

Currently, EU MRLs are replacing UK MRLs. About 280 active substances are now approved for use as agricultural pesticides in the UK, and around 680 are approved in one or more EU states. In 2003, in the UK, over 3,500 samples of food were collected from retail outlets and tested. In addition, DEFRA inspectors collected 500 samples from ports, wholesalers, import points and retail depots. Where there is wide seasonal variation in the source of supply, as is the case for most fruit and vegetables, samples were collected each month for the whole year. Of the total of 4,071 food samples analysed in 2003, no residues at all were found in 75 per cent of them. Residues below the MRL were found in 24 per cent of the samples. In less than 1 per cent of the samples, the residues exceeded the MRL.

In all, the Pesticide Residue Committee has reported the results for over 170,000 pesticide/commodity combinations. As part of the violation investigation programme, fruit and vegetables coming from a source where the produce has exceeded the MRLs in the past are targeted for special attention. When a crop is found in which the pesticide-residue level exceeds the MRL, it is seized and destroyed.

Illness due to pesticide residues is exceedingly rare and mostly confined to countries without well-developed regulatory systems, or to accidents. In spite of this, it has been suggested that sporadic cases of poisoning might easily be missed or misdiagnosed. It is reassuring that, among the thousands of publications relating to the toxicity of organophosphorus insecticides, a search of all the relevant literature has not revealed a single incident that has been associated with residues marginally exceeding MRLs.

The main problem with pesticides remains one of the contamination of foodstuffs used in large amounts in the preparation of meals, either during preparation, storage or transportation. This is almost exclusively a problem of their uncontrolled use in the developing world. These two scenarios – one relating to residues, the other to contamination – are separate and should not be confused. The regulatory mechanisms for monitoring pesticide residue in fruit and vegetables in developed countries are as robust and thorough as possible. They operate with a large margin of safety and are constantly being reviewed to ensure that consumers of any age can eat as much fruit and vegetables as they like without any fear of ill health due to pesticides.

Chapter Fourteen

VITAMINS, MINERALS AND OTHER SUPPLEMENTS

BY DAVID A BENDER

The Myth: **Vitamin supplements promote good health.**

The Fact: **Many supplements supply vitamins in what could be dangerously high doses.**

Almost half the population of Britain takes supplements, spending nearly £400 million a year, and the market is growing. Healthy adults use supplements either because they believe that modern foods are nutrient-depleted or to promote 'optimum health', which may be defined as current well-being and maximum resistance to future infectious and degenerative diseases. Some people take high-dose supplements in the belief that they may confer specific health benefits, for example reducing the risk of developing cancer or heart disease.

Many convenience foods are high in fat and sugars, and relatively poor in vitamins and minerals – they have a low nutrient density, which is the content of vitamins and minerals expressed per 1,000 calories. However, it is not correct to say that the ingredients from which these foods are made are nutrient-depleted. There is no evidence that foods produced by conventional or intensive agriculture are any richer or poorer in nutrients than those produced by traditional or organic farming. Sometimes the varieties grown by organic farmers naturally have a higher nutrient content than some other, possibly higher-yielding, varieties, but the vitamin content of fruits and vegetables varies considerably, depending not only on the variety but also on the growing conditions and stage of ripeness. Apples from one side of the tree may have a very different vitamin content from those on the other side. The mineral content will depend more on the mineral content of the soil, and any fertilisers used, than anything else. Nevertheless, people whose diet consists largely of low-nutrient-density foods may well have an inadequate intake of vitamins and minerals, and may benefit from supplements.

Our estimates of vitamin requirements and tables of recommended or reference intakes are amounts that are calculated to ensure that no one suffers from deficiency. Reference intakes are derived on the basis of the average requirement for a given population group, plus twice the standard deviation around that requirement. This means that they are higher than the requirements of almost everyone in the population. Average intakes of most vitamins and minerals in developed countries are above the reference intakes, and certainly deficiency disease is extremely rare among healthy people. The exception here is iron: many women have greater losses of iron because of menstrual blood loss than can be met from foods, and women generally have very low iron reserves compared to men. Mild iron-deficiency anaemia is not uncommon in premenopausal women, and supplements are needed.

The problem is the definition of the word *requirement*. It is not too difficult to determine a level of intake that will ensure that people do not show any of the subtle biochemical signs of inadequacy, and have adequate body reserves. It is very much more difficult to determine levels of intake that will promote optimum health, which in itself is difficult to define – it is certainly not simply lack of disease. Unfortunately, experiments to determine appropriate levels of intake to maintain optimum health and quality of life into old age will, of necessity, take many years to conduct. There are a number of promising suggestions for metabolic markers of free-radical damage, immune responses and damage to DNA that can be used to determine requirements, but we do not yet know how far these so-called 'biomarkers' reflect the likelihood of developing chronic degenerative diseases such as heart disease, cancer, Parkinsonism or Alzheimer's disease. None of the biomarkers is responsive to only a single nutrient, and all are affected by many non-nutritional factors. To date, we do not have any markers that can be used to determine optimum or protective intakes.

The important questions are whether levels of vitamin and mineral intake higher than current reference intakes may provide health benefits, and whether high intakes are safe.

ARE THERE BENEFITS FROM HIGHER LEVELS OF INTAKE?

A number of epidemiological studies have produced evidence that people whose intake of specific vitamins and minerals is higher than average, or whose blood levels and body reserves of nutrients are high, are less likely to suffer from heart disease and some cancers. This has led to large-scale intervention trials, in which a group of people are given supplements (commonly for 5–15 years) and their medical history, disease incidence and death are compared with a matched population who do not receive the supplements. In general, these intervention trials have been disappointing. The underlying problem is that the people not taking supplements may nevertheless have a high intake of vitamins and minerals, or a high blood level of a specific nutrient, as a result of a high consumption of fruit and vegetables. These contain a wide variety of potentially protective compounds, not only the vitamin or mineral of current interest. Also, a diet that is high in fruit and vegetables is likely to be lower in fat, and especially saturated fat, which in itself is a significant factor in the development of heart disease and some cancers.

Vitamin E and Beta-carotene

There is clear epidemiological evidence that people with a high plasma concentration of vitamin E are less at risk from atherosclerosis and heart disease. Intervention studies have not shown any significant benefit from vitamin E supplements: in one large-scale study in the UK there was a reduction in non-fatal heart attacks, but no decrease or even a small increase in fatal heart attacks and death from all causes. While there are obvious benefits from reducing non-fatal attacks, this is hardly convincing evidence of the benefits of vitamin E supplements. More worryingly, a review of all published trials of vitamin E supplementation showed that people taking relatively high-dose supplements were more likely to die prematurely than those not taking the supplements.

There is also clear epidemiological evidence that high intakes, and high blood levels, of beta-carotene are associated with lower incidence of lung, prostate and other cancers. In a study in China, supplements of beta-carotene, vitamin E and selenium given to a marginally malnourished population led to a reduction in mortality from a variety of cancers. However, a 12-year trial of beta-carotene supplements in the USA showed no effect on the incidence of heart disease or cancer. The results of two major intervention studies with beta-carotene, one in Finland among smokers and the other in the USA among people who had been exposed to asbestos, both yielded unexpected, and unwanted, results – more people receiving the supposedly protective supplements died from lung (and other) cancer than those receiving placebo.

Both vitamin E and beta-carotene are antioxidants and might be expected to reduce the free-radical damage that underlies the development of both cancer and cardiovascular disease. However, most compounds that act as antioxidants do so by forming stable radicals that persist long enough to undergo metabolism to non-radical compounds. By definition they therefore form radicals that can penetrate deeper into tissues and plasma lipoproteins, and potentially cause more damage than the oxygen radicals they have replaced.

Vitamin C

Vitamin C is an antioxidant, and also inhibits the formation of carcinogenic nitrosamines from dietary amines and nitrites. It might therefore be expected to have protective action against the development of cancer and cardiovascular disease. The epidemiological evidence linking a high intake of vitamin C with reduced cancer incidence is confounded by the fact that the fruits and vegetables that are sources of vitamin C are also rich in a variety of other protective compounds. Studies of biomarkers of oxidative damage to DNA have not provided evidence of a protective effect of vitamin C, except in people whose habitual intake was low.

High doses of vitamin C are popularly recommended for the prevention and treatment of the common cold. The results of controlled trials are unconvincing: there is little or no evidence that high intakes of vitamin C reduce the incidence of colds. There is, however, evidence from many studies of a beneficial effect in reducing the severity and duration of symptoms, although this is a notoriously difficult subject to research.

Vitamin D and Calcium

An intake of vitamin D above the amount that can be obtained from normal diets (possibly in combination with supplementary calcium) delays the loss of bone with increasing age, so supplements may be advisable to prevent, or slow the progression of, osteoporosis and osteomalacia. Certainly, there is good evidence that a high intake of calcium in adolescence and young adulthood leads to greater bone density, and therefore delays the development of osteoporosis and osteomalacia in old age. Normal sunlight exposure may provide the equivalent of 20–50 µg/day (considerably above average intakes from foods), so, for most people, increased sunlight exposure may be more effective than supplements, although we have to balance the beneficial effects on bone against increased risk of skin cancer. There are few dietary sources of vitamin D, and supplements are recommended for the housebound elderly who have little exposure to sunlight.

Folic Acid

The benefits of folic-acid supplements taken before and during pregnancy in preventing spina bifida and other neural-tube defects have been demonstrated convincingly, and women planning pregnancy are advised to take supplements of 400 µg of folic acid per day – this is more than twice the reference intake, and could not be achieved without the use of supplements. High intakes of folic acid (again above the amount that could be obtained from normal diets) lower plasma homocysteine, which is a genetically determined risk factor for heart disease and stroke, and low intakes of folic acid are associated with increased risk of colo-rectal cancer. As yet there are no results from intervention trials to determine whether supplements of folic acid will reduce death from heart disease and stroke, or the incidence of colo-rectal cancer.

In the USA and a number of other countries, fortification of flour with folic acid is required by law, but it is too soon to know whether this will affect the incidence of neural-tube defects, heart disease or cancer.

Vitamin B6

Many women take supplements of vitamin B_6 of the order of 50–200 milligrams per day (compared with a reference intake of 1.5–2 milligrams) to treat premenstrual syndrome. There is little evidence from controlled trials that it is effective, and the safety of high intakes of vitamin B_6 has been questioned. There is good evidence that intakes in excess of 500 milligrams per day lead to nerve damage, which may be only partly reversed on ceasing the supplementation. However, there is little or no evidence that intakes of up to 200 milligrams per day have any adverse effects.

Vitamin B12

Vitamin B_{12} is found only in foods of animal origin, or as a result of bacterial contamination of foods, and strict vegetarians (or vegans) have a negligible intake, so are indeed well advised to take supplements prepared by bacterial fermentation which are ethically acceptable to them. Vitamin B_{12} deficiency can also develop as a result of progressive loss of secretion of gastric juice with increasing age, leading to impaired absorption of the vitamin from foods. Again, supplements are advisable in such cases, especially since high intakes of folic acid (from supplements or fortified cereals) can mask the development of anaemia due to vitamin B_{12} deficiency, but do not protect against the irreversible nerve damage.

There have been reports of vegans developing vitamin B_{12} deficiency because they have eaten plant foods (including algae such as spirulina and seaweed, and fermented soya products such as tofu) believing them to contain vitamin B_{12}, and have not taken supplements. Unfortunately, what is present in these foods is a compound related to vitamin B_{12} that supports the growth of the micro-organisms used for the standard method of measuring vitamin B_{12} in foods, but is not active as the vitamin in human beings. There have been some reports of algae containing biologically active vitamin B_{12}, but this varies depending on the source of the algae, and it is likely that it is due to contamination of lakes with faecal bacteria that synthesise the vitamin.

Selenium

Selenium is required as part of the body's antioxidant defences, and there is good evidence from China and other areas of the world where selenium deficiency is common that supplementation, food fortification or use of selenium-containing fertilisers reduces the incidence of various cancers. There is concern in the UK that average intakes of selenium have fallen by almost half over the last 20 years, mainly as a result of using wheat grown in Europe, where the soil is relatively poor in selenium, rather than wheat grown in North America and Australia, where soils are richer in selenium. There is, however, little evidence that selenium supplements have any beneficial effect at current average European intakes, and, more worryingly, the margin between an adequate intake of selenium and the level at which signs of toxicity develop is very small.

Fluoride

There is overwhelming evidence that people in areas where the drinking water contains about one part per million of fluoride suffer considerably less dental decay than those whose intake of fluoride is lower. This has led to the deliberate fluoridation of water in many areas, with a resultant decrease in dental decay. However, fluoridation of water is an emotive subject, and many people regard it as compulsory 'mass medication'. For people whose water is poor in fluoride, supplements (and the use of fluoride-containing toothpaste and mouthwash) are probably advisable. However, in areas where the fluoride content of water is above about 10 parts per million there are problems of fluoride toxicity – dark mottling of the teeth may be only a cosmetic problem, but at these high levels of intake there are also problems of changes in bone mineralisation, leading to increased bone fragility and greater susceptibility to fractures. This has led to warnings about the use of fluoride supplements and fluoride-containing toothpaste and mouthwashes.

Fish-oil Supplements

There is good evidence from both epidemiological and intervention studies that the fatty acids in fish oil (the omega-3 series of polyunsaturated fatty acids) are protective against atherosclerosis and heart disease, and may also be beneficial in treating osteoarthritis and enhancing immune-system function. The general advice is that people should eat one or two meals of oily fish each week, but some people do not like fish, or are concerned about mercury pollution in wild salmon and tuna, and organic pesticides in farmed salmon and trout. Supplements of cod- and other fish-liver oil are available as a source of omega-3 polyunsaturated fatty acids.

Bodybuilding Supplements

There is a bewildering array of other supplements on the market. Some are traditional herbal remedies, others are ingredients in so-called functional foods – foods that provide some additional health benefit, or supplements containing nutrients other than vitamins and minerals – and others are single amino acids or mixed-protein supplements. Some, especially those sold for bodybuilding, also contain stimulants and potentially harmful anabolic steroids. Increasingly, supplements that contain illegal substances are being sold over the Internet where there is no regulation and no redress for the consumer should there be adverse effects. Similarly, Internet advertising may contain misleading claims that might well be illegal in more conventional advertising, and would form the basis of prosecution by trading-standards officers if it weren't for the fact that no one has jurisdiction over the Internet, and dishonest traders cannot readily be prosecuted.

THE SAFETY OF HIGH INTAKES OF VITAMINS AND MINERALS

Vitamins and minerals are considered to be foods, and their sale is therefore regulated by food laws. This means that, when high intakes of vitamins are recommended for the treatment or prevention of diseases, the consumer has little protection. High-dose supplements are freely available from a variety of outlets – pharmacies, supermarkets and 'health-food' stores. There is an argument that supplement sales should be regulated, with doses of up to (say) three to five times the reference intake being freely available, but higher doses to be sold only by pharmacists who are qualified to give medicinal advice. Some argue that higher doses, where there is a possibility of adverse effects, should be available only on prescription, since qualified medical practitioners are specifically trained to consider the risk/benefit balance of treatments. The counter-argument is that there should be no restriction on sales unless there is evidence of a toxic hazard – the consumer should be free to decide.

Vitamins A, D, B_6 and niacin are all known to be toxic in excess, as are many minerals. The intake at which the toxic effects of vitamin A occurs is about 10–12 times the reference intake for adults, and about three times the reference intake for infants. Some children develop hypercalcaemia and calcinosis as a result of vitamin D intakes as low as 45 µg/day, compared with a reference intake of 5–10 µg.

Various government reports on reference intakes provide guidance about prudent upper limits of habitual consumption of vitamins and minerals, and the US/Canadian reports have established tolerable upper limits for many. The tolerable upper level is defined as the maximum level of habitual intake that is unlikely to pose any risk of adverse health effects to almost all individuals in the stated population group. It is a level of intake that can (with a high degree of probability) be tolerated biologically, but is not a recommended level and, according to the US Institute of Medicine, 'there is no established benefit for healthy individuals consuming more than the reference daily requirement'.

In the UK, the Foods Standards Agency set up the Expert Group on Vitamins and Minerals 'to establish principles on which controls for ensuring the safety of vitamin and mineral supplements sold under food law can be based; to review the levels of individual vitamins and minerals associated with adverse effects; and to recommend maximum levels of intakes of vitamins and minerals from supplements if appropriate'. It has published a series of working documents evaluating the evidence of safety or hazard, from which upper levels of safe intake can be determined.

The European Federation of Health Food Manufacturers has published upper limits of vitamins and minerals for use in over-the-counter supplements; although these are voluntary, responsible manufacturers are likely to abide by them. Problems may arise when people consume supplements made by less responsible manufacturers, who may have poor control over the amount of the vitamins or minerals in their products. Equally, problems may arise when people take a variety of different supplements, each of which contains only the safe upper limit, but the combination may provide an unsafe amount.

NATURAL VERSUS SYNTHETIC VITAMINS

Some people believe that natural-source vitamins are superior to chemically synthesised vitamins. In most cases, this is not true – the synthetic vitamin is identical to the naturally occurring material, and has exactly the same biological action. There are two exceptions: vitamin E and folic acid.

Naturally occurring vitamin E is a mixture of eight different compounds, each with different potency – the most potent is alpha-tocopherol. Alpha-tocopherol has complex stereochemistry, and the different stereo-isomers have different potencies. Natural-source alpha-tocopherol consists solely of the most potent isomer, all-R-alpha-tocopherol, while the synthetic material is a mixture of the different isomers. This means that natural-source vitamin E is more potent than the synthetic vitamin.

With folic acid the reverse is true. There are various forms of folic acid in foods (collectively called food folates), and these are digested and absorbed to different extents. By contrast, synthetic folic acid, as used in supplements and food fortification, consists of a single chemical compound, the most readily absorbed and utilised form. As a result, synthetic folic acid is some 1.4 times more potent than the mixed folates found in unfortified foods.

HERBAL REMEDIES

A number of modern pharmaceuticals have been derived from naturally occurring compounds in various herbs, many of which have long been used by medical herbalists and in traditional medicine. While some traditional and herbal remedies are effective, there is little evidence of the efficacy, or indeed safety, of many. Preparations such as ginseng, ginkgo biloba and other herbal supplements contain pharmacologically active compounds, many of which interact with prescribed medication, either enhancing or reducing its efficacy. Unfortunately, few people think of such supplements as medication, considering them to be 'natural' and therefore perceiving them as safe, and so do not mention them to doctors when they are asked what other medication they are taking. This can have potentially serious effects.

There are two further problems with herbal remedies. Very few have been subjected to rigorous controlled testing for efficacy or safety. Indeed, it is unlikely that many ever will be tested for efficacy, since proper controlled trials are extremely expensive. With prescription medication, the costs of development and testing can be recovered from sales while the drug is under patent, but for herbal remedies there is no patent protection, and hence no period of time during which an adequate profit can be made to recoup the costs of testing.

The second problem is one of quality control and the standardisation of preparations. Larger and more responsible manufacturers have adequate laboratory facilities to ensure the quality and potency of their products; many smaller companies do not, and the potency (and even safety) of their products may differ widely from one batch to another.

Unfortunately, since supplements are sold under food laws rather than the laws governing medicines, there is little regulation of the market, and the consumer has little protection against snake-oil vendors, quacks and charlatans. In the UK, anyone who considers that he or she has been misled by advertising can ask the local trading-standards officer to investigate and bring a prosecution under the Sale of Goods Act. Such prosecutions are difficult, however, since it can be difficult to counter vague, unscientific arguments with precise cautious science. While a scientist may understand the difference between a properly conducted randomised controlled trial and uncontrolled 'trials' and experiments, if the latter have been published (albeit hopefully not in a peer-reviewed medical or scientific journal), it can be difficult to persuade a magistrate who is not a trained scientist. Equally, some of the less reputable manufacturers and suppliers fail to appear in court, then move their business to another county under the jurisdiction of a different local authority's trading-standards officer, so evading prosecution until another officer can be persuaded to take action.

FUNCTIONAL FOODS

A number of foods are now available that contain ingredients intended to have specific health-promoting effects. Examples include yoghurts containing live cultures of bacteria that are intended to colonise the large intestine with 'friendly' bacteria and displace potentially pathogenic bacteria – so-called bio-yoghurts. Some foods contain carbohydrates that are not digested in the small intestine, but pass to the colon where they provide nutrition for desirable intestinal bacteria. There is some evidence that both probiotics (live bacterial cultures) and prebiotics (the compounds that nourish 'friendly bacteria') are beneficial, although it is uncertain how long colonisation of the large intestine with probiotics lasts unless you continue to consume the yoghurt.

Two groups of compounds used in (expensive) yoghurt, margarine and other dairy produce, plant sterols and stanol esters are chemically similar to cholesterol and inhibit its absorption from the small intestine. Average intakes of cholesterol from the diet are around 0.5 grams per day, but we secrete about two grams of cholesterol in the bile each day, most of which is normally reabsorbed. There is very good evidence that these compounds, together with a prudent diet, reduce serum cholesterol significantly, so avoiding the need for cholesterol-lowering medication in many people.

Sugar is a well-know cause of dental decay, and a number of manufacturers produce sweets and chewing gum containing the 5-carbon sugar alcohol xylitol. A number of controlled trials have shown that xylitol specifically inhibits the growth of plaque-forming bacteria in the mouth, and so acts to prevent tooth decay. Such sweets are commonly marketed as being 'tooth-friendly'.

CONCLUSION

There are some cases where there is evidence that intakes of vitamins and minerals over and above what can be obtained from food may be beneficial, and some people with a poor diet may need supplements; but in general there is little evidence that supplements are beneficial, and in some cases they may provide dangerously high levels of intake.

Chapter Fifteen

FOOD ADDITIVES:
HOW SAFE, HOW VALUABLE?

BY MAURICE HANSSEN

'E for Additives (M. Hanssen)'

OXFORD ENGLISH DICTIONARY

The Myth: **E numbers are harmful and undesirable.**
The Fact: **Most E numbers are perfectly safe, and their use is well controlled.**

A survey by the British Consumer Association in 2004 found that a third of people try to avoid food additives for fear of adverse effects on their health. It is true that some additives can cause problems for a few of us, and that it is now possible to disguise a product in such a way that, although it is very high in fats and water and contains little of nutritional worth, it tastes delicious and fools our senses into believing that it is good for us.

It is equally true that the modern food-supply chain could not exist without food additives. We are blessed with foods that can be very safe and stay fresh for a longer time than ever before.

Additives have been used for thousands of years. Today, almost all wines have added sulphites to prevent them going off or fermenting. Some asthmatics find that this can trigger an attack but, like the ancient Greeks who burned sulphur over their amphorae of wine to produce sulphites, we just enjoy the fruits of the vine. After November 2005 it will be necessary to declare the presence of sulphites (E221–8), as California has done for many years. Medieval chefs decorated their elaborate confections of marzipan with bright colours to entrance the senses – gold and silver (E175 and E174) have been used to decorate confectionary and festive dishes throughout recorded history. Our ancestors well understood the preservative properties of salting and smoking and also curing meats with saltpetre (E252) and brine to provide meat and fish throughout the year.

The industrial revolution brought in the roller milling of wheat to produce white flour but, in an effort to make flour whiter, some unscrupulous millers added white lead, thought to have caused more deaths than influenza in the nineteenth century. Such abuses were brought to light by a Jewish/Huguenot chemist, Frederick Carl Accum. In 1820, he published 'A Treatise on Adulterations of Food and Culinary Poisons'. This was a devastating exposé of many dangerous practices of the time. The preface reminded readers that, 'However invidious the office may appear, and however painful the duty may be, of exposing the names of individuals who have been convicted of adulterating food, yet it was necessary for the verification of my statement.' The UK Food Standards Agency wisely adopts the same policy today.

In spite of Accum, it was not until public pressure forced the government to enact the Food Labelling Regulations of 1984 that manufacturers began the disclosure of ingredients including additives. This became mandatory on 1 January 1986, and the letter E – standing for European numbers – was designated for a wide range of additives, which steadily grows, giving us a list that now identifies some 320 substances.

The identification of illegal additives in foods is as important today as in Victorian times. The difficulty is this: how do you find a substance that you do not expect to be there? We expect – and look out for – preservatives in sausages, and can check to see if they are at legal levels;

but antifreeze in wine? In July 1984, an enquiring Austrian VAT inspector wondered why a winery was claiming back VAT on significant quantities of diethylene glycol antifreeze in the summer. He had uncovered the Austrian wine scandal: adding this antifreeze makes cheap wines taste like top-class vintages, but unfortunately a daily intake of just 3 millilitres – or half a teaspoon – is enough to cause kidney damage, and 100 millilitres is fatal. A bottle bought in Barnsley of one of the 82 implicated brands contained 1.5 millilitres, so a heavy drinker would be at substantial risk.

More recently, in 2004, the Food Standards Agency reported on products, mostly from India, that contained the potentially carcinogenic red colour Sudan 1. By the end of the year they had identified lists of products occupying eight closely crowded pages. These included curry and tandoori mixes, jerk seasoning, chilli and tomato sauces and relishes, chutneys, pesto, couscous and balsamic-vinegar-based sauces to mention but a few. Luckily, the tip of an iceberg was discovered and the investigations that followed yielded results which shamed many distinguished brands.

However, E does not stand for Evil or Evade. E numbers provide the information upon which we can make informed choices, be they on environmental, ethical, gastronomic or health grounds. With hindsight, the labelling requirement that allows additives to be described either by the E number or the chemical name has made life less easy for the consumer. Often the two are mixed, making the named additives look more like normal ingredients, so confusion still persists. For example, children's drinks often describe E102 as tartrazine because E102 is known to precipitate hyperactivity in a few children, but put E300, which is ascorbic acid, on the label as the number.

When I wrote my book *E for Additives* in 1984, I found that I had a problem with less than one in five additives; more than two decades later, there is a significant reduction in the use of some additives which can cause intolerances or adverse effects in small, but significant, groups of people. My concerns are now towards the many foods aimed at children and the less well-off which are close to nutritional rubbish.

Aspartame (NutraSweet) has been attacked, mostly by activists in the USA, as being harmful. I am sure this is a false judgement based on non-scientific evidence. The campaigning against aspartame resulted in the substance being reassessed by the EU Scientific Committee on Food in 2002. They decided it was safe. Sweeteners are given a very rigorous examination by regulators because, unlike the majority of additives, they may well be used every day for many years.

The point has been well made earlier in this book that toxicity is dose-related – drink nine litres of water in half an hour and you will probably die. Any additive or ingredient in excess can be harmful: this is why ADIs (Acceptable Daily Intakes) are assessed for many additives by the Joint Expert Committee on Food Additives (JECFA), which are translated into EU levels by the European Food Safety Authority (EFSA).

Additives are grouped into six general categories according to their purposes. Labels have to define the use before stating the numbers. You might read, 'colours E102, E110, preservatives E211, E220'. Just as ingredients are listed in descending order by weight or volume, so are the additives. This is valuable information which helps you make an informed decision about the food when you read the label. The link to the Food Standards Agency list of European Union-approved additives can be found at:
www.food.gov.uk/safereating/additivesbranch/enumberlist.

COLOURS

There are 44 colours, numbered from E100 (Curcumin, an extract of yellow turmeric) to E180 (Litholrubine, a reddish azo dye that is safe).

Azo colours have a molecular configuration, which means that some of them produce adverse reactions in sensitive, allergic people, especially asthmatics, those with eczema and the aspirin-sensitive. These can cause nettle rash, wheezing and watering of the eyes or nose. They are E102, E110, E122, E123, E124, E128, E151, E154, E155 and E180.

Coal-tar colours used to be derived from coal and were discovered by Sir William Perkins in 1856. They revolutionised the dyeing of cloth. Some coal-tar dyes are also azo colours. They include the above plus E104, E127, E131, E132 and E133. Some of these colours have been implicated in hyperactivity in children. It has been suggested that avoiding them can control this serious problem when combined with a good diet, without the potential side-effects of putting young people on to strong drugs such as Ritalin.

Many other colours have a long history of safe use, and indeed coal-tar and azo dyes are harmless for the vast majority.

PRESERVATIVES

There are 39 preservatives used to avoid some foods deteriorating and to prevent food poisoning. They number from sorbic acid E200, which occurs naturally in the berries of the mountain ash and which inhibits yeast and mould growths in unpasteurised cheeses and milk products, to borax E285, plus lysozyme E1105. Benzoic acid E210, which occurs naturally in many berries, fruits and vegetables along with the colour tartrazine E102, provoked an adverse response in 27 out of 34 hyperactive children.

On any risk/benefit assessment of the preservatives, the risk to most of us is very low and the benefits considerable.

ANTIOXIDANTS

The 15 antioxidants number from ascorbic acid E300 (which is vitamin C) to butylated hydroxytoluene (BHT) E321. When we cut open an apple, the flesh goes brown because it has oxidised. If, as soon as we cut it, we add lemon juice – which contains both natural E300 and citric acid E330, which enhances its effect – then freshness is preserved for some time.

Some antioxidants, such as E300, are best at preserving non-fatty foods, whereas E306–9 are all forms of vitamin E which can stop fats going rancid. They are very safe; indeed, it is an advantage when cooking oils contain natural or added vitamin E, especially if they are in clear glass bottles, as light encourages oxidation; in an ideal world, oils and milk would be sold in opaque containers.

The last two in the list, E320 and 321 – BHA and BHT – have pros and cons ranging from a possible reduction of cancers in some people to a negative effect in others. On the whole they are safe, but it is probably wise to limit consumption by young children. They are used in some high-calorie fatty foods.

SWEETENERS

It is with sweeteners that the logic in the numbering system breaks down. The 16 sweeteners start with sorbitol E420, which used to be popular in diabetic foods but, as it is half as sweet as sugar and has a similar calorie content, it has now fallen out of favour. It is used in many filled chocolates and confectionary as it helps keep the contents moist in the mouth and prevents the formation of crystals. The remaining sweeteners include: mannitol E421, which occurs in nature with similar properties to sorbitol but has fewer calories; lactitol E966; xylitol E967, a sweetener originally derived from the silver birch which is now often used in chewing gum because it helps prevent tooth decay while being sweet; E951 aspartame is safe and tastes good without the bitter aftertaste of E954 saccharine. Two sweeteners were added in 2003: sucralose, E955, which is 600 times sweeter than sugar and is marketed as Splenda, and E962 salt of aspartame-acesulfame. It is likely that another sweetener, E968 erythritol, will soon be approved.

One of the reasons we have so many sweeteners is that different processes and acidities need appropriate sweeteners to make the food product palatable. It is a competitive market subject to many individual preferences.

EMULSIFIERS, STABILISERS, THICKENERS AND GELLING AGENTS

These 60 additives from E322 to E495, plus invertase E1103, have technical functions ranging from mixing oil and water, such as the first, lecithins E322, which is in all our bodily cells and is found in high concentrations in soya beans and egg yolk, to thickeners like guar gum E412, which allows emulsions and thickened foods to stay in suspension to give body to the product. It is a safe group of useful additives with the exception of the misuse of the gums, especially guar and konjac E425, when sucked in sweets or in capsules. If these stick in the throat, they expand greatly and have caused death by asphyxiation. Such products are now banned.

There is a major commercial issue with the group of E450 additives, the perfectly safe polyphosphates. These additives enable the producer to combine large quantities of water with, for example, meat and ham. That is why much bacon turns into a salty slurry in the pan and canned hams are routinely found with 30 per cent added water. These additions are rarely reflected in a lower price.

OTHERS

There are 135 remaining additives, and they are largely self-explanatory. They include: acids, acidity regulators, anti-caking agents, anti-foaming agents, bulking agents, carriers and carrier solvents, emulsifying salts, firming agents, flavour enhancers, flour-treatment agents, foaming agents, glazing agents, humectants, modified starches, packaging gases, propellants, raising agents and sequestrants.

This catch-everything-else group of 135 additives with a selection of numbers from E170, calcium carbonate, or chalk, used for firming some canned fruits and vegetables and in food supplements, to E1520, Propylene glycol. This is used as a carrier and carrier solvent in colours, emulsifiers, antioxidants and enzymes.

These additives are technical aids with functions such as to improve the texture or appearance, to improve the flavour, to pressurise aerosols, to make bread and cake mixes rise and to provide protective atmospheres so that oxygen cannot spoil fresh foods such as fish, meat and fruit. This group of gases such as E938, Argon, E939, Helium and E 941, Nitrogen, are a boon to once-a-week shoppers enabling perishable products to survive in the refrigerator far better than their ungassed equivalents.

There has been a lot of debate about the flavour enhancer E621, monosodium glutamate. With the proviso that we can all be allergic or sensitive to something, MSG is a valuable, safe ingredient. It has been linked to a supposed condition known as 'Chinese-restaurant syndrome'. This was said to cause a selection of symptoms ranging from numbness of the neck to headaches and palpitations. Sufferers were given different drinks with and without MSG, and showed the symptoms each time!

I have checked in Chinese takeaways and some were using a heaped teaspoon in every portion. This is bad practice and will in any case give you far too much sodium. Use the tail of the spoon.

The glutamate story is that since time immemorial Japanese cooks have used the seaweed *laminaria japonica* to improve and bring out the flavour of foods cooked in savoury stocks. In 1908 Tokyo professor Kikunae Ikeda isolated the active substance, glutamic acid. It was found that we have separate taste buds to the usual sweet, sour, salt and bitter, which detect and appreciate glutamates. The taste was called *umami* which means 'deliciousness'.

It is one of the mechanisms which bond babies to mothers because their milk contains 22 mg glutamate per 100 ml, 10 times as much as cow's milk. Tomatoes and parmesan cheese are also naturally rich in glutamates, hence our love of pizzas and the valuable additive E621!

FLAVOURS

The European Union is engaged on a long-term project to validate the safety and quality of the 3,000 flavours in current use, often added in combinations of 10 or 20 varieties to achieve the desired result. It seems unlikely that there is space on most labels to list a separate set of numbers and, as adverse effects are almost unknown, it is probably not needed. They can be natural as in vanilla or nature identical as in vanillin, its key flavour component, as well as synthetic. They can be described on the label as 'flavouring' but many producers describe tastes that are artificial as, for example, 'banana flavour' when there is no banana present and as 'banana flavoured' when there is.

Additives are desirable and useful when used in the right way. They are essential to modern food processing and some have a very long history. Abuses are possible and there is no doubt that certain groups of people can be allergic or intolerant to some additives including colours and preservatives. The E-number system allows us to make informed choices. There is no substitute for always reading the label and enjoying the food.

Chapter Sixteen

FOOD LABELLING

BY STANLEY FELDMAN

The Myth: Food labelling allows us to make informed choices about all the food and drink we consume.

The Fact: Labelling is not applied uniformly and in the case of fresh produce is not applied at all.

We used to eat food that we liked and drink water that came straight from the tap. Today we are told what we should eat and what we should avoid. Unless we follow the instructions from these self-styled experts we are threatened with heart attacks, diabetes, sterility, cancer and premature death.

Tap water is out of fashion and a huge industry has appeared to persuade us to drink bottled water, much of which starts out coming from the same source as the tap water that we no longer trust. The consumer is now the victim of the very system that was set up to protect him.

I have in front of me a bottle of 'pure water'. It has on its reverse side a list of 10 ingredients other than water. On further inspection, none of these is in a concentration that is harmful, and even at 100 times their concentration I doubt it would cause any ill effect if I drank the whole bottle at one go. All are naturally occurring chemicals. I am not influenced by this list of contents. I drink that particular water because it quenches my thirst and I like the taste. If the bottle were filled with tap water, this too would require a list of the minute amounts of harmless chemicals it contains. However, if I take the water straight from the tap no labelling is necessary, although the concentration of the minute amounts of chemicals will vary according to the region where the water originated. Labelling of this kind serves no purpose at all. None of the chemicals it contains will harm us in the concentrations present. The one thing I would really like to know is the concentration of the bacteria E. coli. Although in itself not dangerous, indeed our bowels are crawling with these bacteria, a high bacterial count does indicate the likelihood of faecal contamination of the water and could lead to illness. All water, whether bottled or not, contains E. coli in concentrations that are harmless to us. In fact, *Which* magazine did an investigation that showed the so-called 'natural waters' generally had a higher E. coli count than those made up from tap water.

This one potentially important piece of information, which would indicate the purity of the product, is not listed so why list chemicals that will do us no harm at all and not list bacteria that might? Food labelling has lost its way. It no longer serves to warn the consumer of potential dangers or health risks; it has become a marketing gimmick.

If we were left to our own devices we would select the food we eat and the fluid we drink because we liked the taste; it assuages our hunger and provides the necessary energy and nutriment to sustain life. We would not choose what foods to eat on the basis of its chemical analysis. The purpose of labelling is to make sure we are not misled, our health is not put at risk and we can choose one product in preference to another. Instead, it has become a device that confuses the consumer and can be used to conceal information. It has become mandatory to display the list of contents on all processed foods regardless of how helpful this list is. We do not label the content of non-processed food, such as a lamb chop, a banana or a walnut, although all of these have contents that vary greatly according to how it has been produced and which, in excess, can be harmful to some people. A kipper contains a high concentration of salt but does not require labelling until it is put in a bag when it becomes 'a processed food'. We expect a kipper to be salty and it does not change when it is put into a bag; we eat it as part of a balanced diet because we like the taste or believe it does us good.

The reasoning behind the consumer pressure for the lists of content to be displayed on processed food is that it allows us to make an informed choice in selecting those foods we are told are good for us and in rejecting those containing substances we are told are bad. The pressure to make us all eat food that so-called experts think is 'healthy' and the resulting consumer anxiety over identifying 'healthy food' has led to the suggestion that foods should be 'traffic lighted', colour-coded according to how much salt, sugar or fat they contain. A green mark would indicate food we should 'eat plenty' of, while a red mark would indicate food we should avoid. It is difficult to see the benefits of such a daft system even if it could be consistently applied. A small packet of sweets would be labelled as bad because it may contain a lot of sugar which is fattening, while a large bag of the same sweets containing less sugar but with added saccharine would be good. An apple would be good yet it is possible that it may contain more sugar than some sweets. How would they label a can of Coca-Cola, which contains slightly less calories than a similar-sized can of orange juice? Salads would be labelled as a 'good food' but, once they are covered in a salad dressing, or salt is added to give them taste, they would become 'bad'. Experience has taught us that 'expert' opinion on what is and is not nutritionally good for us changes. What is good for us one week can be bad the next. What may be given a green before may suddenly change to 'amber' or 'red'. The system could prove more confusing than helpful.

If we rely on labelling to control the amount of certain elements in our diet it can be fraught with difficulty. Having been warned that too much fat in our diet means a heart attack and an early death, we can avoid meat products that are labelled high in fats but meat from a butcher invariably contains fat and is not labelled. A fat content of much less than 10 per cent would make it too tasteless to eat without some oily sauce or flavouring. What do we do about cheese? Buy cheese from the counter of the delicatessen and we are blissfully unaware of its fat content, however shrink-wrapped cheese in the supermarket is required to have a full chemical analysis on the package. Does this mean we must avoid butcher shops and cheese from the counter? It is not what we eat but the amount of it that is important in making people fat.

Food manufacturers should be open and declare when preservatives, colouring or water have been added. However, the producers of the farmed fish, recommended as being a 'good' food, often add colouring to the feed of their fish to improve the way the flesh looks. Unless the fish is packaged for supermarkets, it does not have to have a list of contents. Even smoked food such as ham, which may contain added salt, nitrates and water, does not need to be labelled.

Some foods have water deliberately added, a practice used in the processing of some 'chicken pieces', bacon and turkey. This is not harmful in itself – after all, dry food can be unattractive; a limp cucumber is unpalatable and an apple that has dried out lacks the bite of the fresh fruit. In any event, we invariably drink extra fluid with our meals. We don't worry about the water that makes up about 90 per cent of fresh fruit. Nevertheless, if water is added, then that should be clearly stated and reflected in the price. Without preservatives the shelf life of many foods would be short and the extra cost of the subsequent waste would be an unnecessary burden on the consumer, nevertheless, it is reasonable to expect the addition of a preservative to be indicated on a label of contents.

If a potential allergen, such as peanut oil or gluten, is present in a product, it should be clearly stated so as warn the unwary. The chaotic state of labelling results in prawns being sold without a warning to the consumer, in spite of the high incidence of shellfish allergy; after all, it is what it purports to be, whereas the packs of Scottish smoked salmon from Sainsbury's have to carry a notice that informs me that it contains – surprise surprise – fish.

Go to a health-food shop or a centre of Chinese herbal remedies and one will find pills and potions on sale, many of which contain toxic substances. These potentially dangerous chemicals are unlicensed, untested and uncontrolled and their contents can vary alarmingly, yet they are not required to label their contents. So, while we have a list of harmless ingredients listed on a bottle of water, potentially dangerous toxins contained in a bottle of herbal remedy will not be listed. We should insist these products carrying a health warning where one is necessary. Instead, because they are promoted as 'healthy' and 'natural', they escape legislation. There is an enormous market in these products. It is estimated that 20 per cent of UK adults takes one of these remedies on a regular basis. Those pouring their money into the pockets of these 'snake oil' salesmen should realise that the life expectancy in China is much shorter than the UK in spite of the ready availability of herbal remedies, and that most hospital poison centres regularly treat patients poisoned by such products. The result is a paradox: we have strict legislation requiring the labelling of the contents of the harmless chemicals in water, but fight shy of labelling potentially dangerous herbal remedies.

One of the dangers of the way food is packaged and labelled is that it can be used to fool the consumer. Hamburgers or sausages made of '100 per cent beef' may still contain as little as 50 per cent protein (beef is defined as 'the flesh of cattle'). Not all beef is protein. Products claiming to contain no added sugar may contain a high calorie maple syrup. It only requires one to reduce the fat content of a cheese by 5 per cent to label it 'a low-fat cheese'. A survey for the consumer magazine 'Which' in October 2004 found that some so-called healthy foods contained more saturated fat, sugar or salt than the regular products. It is easy to be seduced by labelling into believing one is eating a healthy diet and forget the dangers of eating too much.

The present system of food labelling is inconsistent. It does not give clear warnings of a potential danger in some fresh foods and as a result it fails to promote the information necessary for a sensible informed choice. At the end of the day, we eat a particular food because it tastes good. No amount of labelling will cajole us into eating food we do not like. Because there is no clear philosophy as to the purpose of listing the contents of food, the system is in a mess. All we should really worry about is that the food we eat is safe, is reasonable value for money and fulfils our nutritional needs and that our total intake roughly matches our bodily requirement.

How many consumers really know the difference between a picogram and a nanogram or what a concentration of 7 parts per 10^7 means? Is there any point in listing these minute concentrations of chemicals? Should the tiny hydrocyanic acid content of almonds be listed? Is it not time to label only those substances that have been added to a food or drink that can harm you in the concentrations actually present, instead of trying to use labelling to change people's lifestyles? Above all, labelling should be consistent, reliable and accurate and should be restricted to substances that may constitute a risk to the health of the consumer.

PART THREE:

HEALTH RISKS?

Chapter Seventeen

THE GREAT CHOLESTEROL MYTH

BY MALCOLM KENDRICK

'For every complicated problem there is a solution that is simple, direct, understandable and wrong.'

HL MENCKEN

The Myth: **A high cholesterol intake causes heart disease.**

The Fact: **Cholesterol levels are not affected by cholesterol intake, and in any case there is no evidence to suggest that cholesterol and heart disease are linked.**

If you eat too much cholesterol, or saturated fat, your blood cholesterol will rise to dangerous levels. Excess cholesterol will then seep through your artery walls causing thickenings (plaques) which will eventually block blood flow in vital arteries, resulting in heart attacks and strokes. Scientific hypotheses don't get much simpler than this, the cholesterol, or diet–heart, hypothesis, which has broken free from the ivory towers of academia to impact with massive force on society.

It has driven a widespread change in the type of food we are told to eat, and consequently the food that lines the supermarket shelves. Many people view bacon and eggs as dangerous killers, butter is shunned and a multi-billion-pound industry has sprung up providing 'healthy' low-fat alternatives.

At the same time, millions of people are prescribed statins to lower cholesterol levels, and each new set of guidelines suggests ever more lowering of cholesterol is needed. When it comes to explaining what causes heart disease, the cholesterol hypothesis reigns supreme.

LANDMARKS IN THE DEVELOPMENT OF THE CHOLESTEROL HYPOTHESIS

1850s: Rudolf Virchow notes the presence of cholesterol in atherosclerotic plaques. Suggests excess cholesterol in the bloodstream may be the cause

Early 1900s: Ashoff feeds rabbits fat and cholesterol, and notes the development of atheroma

1912: First heart attack described by Herrick

1940s: Epidemic of heart disease hits USA, and interest in the area explodes. Many researchers blame high fat/cholesterol diet

1948: The Framingham study on heart disease starts. Still running today

1954: Ancel Key's seminal Seven Countries Study published. Demonstrates clear links between saturated-fat intake and heart disease

1961: Framingham confirms link between raised cholesterol levels and heart disease

1960s: First cholesterol-lowering drugs developed

1970s: Brown and Goldstein find gene leading to extremely high cholesterol levels (familial hypercholesterolaemia) and premature heart disease

1980s: Statins launched

1985:   Nobel Prize for Brown and Goldstein

1990s: Statins trials demonstrate that cholesterol-lowering protects against heart disease

Presented in this way, its not difficult to see how the cholesterol hypothesis became *the* dominant hypothesis, effortlessly kicking alternative ideas into touch. Indeed, to question this theory is to risk being placed on the same shelf as flat-earthers and creationists.

However, all is not what it seems. The cholesterol hypothesis can be likened to a cathedral built on a bog. Rather than admit they made a horrible mistake and let it sink, the builders decided to try and keep the cathedral afloat at all costs. Each time a crack appeared, a new buttress was built. Then further buttresses were built to support the original buttresses. Although direct contradictions to the cholesterol hypothesis repeatedly appear, no one dares say, 'OK, this isn't working, time to build again from scratch.' That decision has become just too painful, especially now that massive industries, Nobel prizes and glittering scientific careers have grown on the back of the cholesterol hypothesis. The statin market alone is worth more than £20 billion each year.

In reality, cracks in the hypothesis appeared right from the very start. The first of these was the stark observation that cholesterol in the diet has no effect on cholesterol levels in the bloodstream:

There's no connection whatsoever between cholesterol in food and cholesterol in blood. And we've known that all along. Cholesterol in the diet doesn't matter at all unless you happen to be a chicken or a rabbit.

ANCEL KEYS, PHD, PROFESSOR EMERITUS AT THE
UNIVERSITY OF MINNESOTA, 1997

A bit of a blow to a cholesterol hypothesis, you might think, to find that dietary cholesterol has no effect on blood cholesterol levels. However, as everyone was, by then, fully convinced that something rich and 'fatty' in the diet was the primary cause of heart disease, no one was willing to let go. So the hypothesis quietly altered from 'cholesterol in the diet' to 'saturated fat in the diet' – or a bit of both, as if, in some way, cholesterol and saturated fat are similar if not almost exactly the same thing.

In reality, this could hardly be further from the truth. Saturated fat and cholesterol have completely different functions in the body, and they have very different chemical structures (see *Figure 3* below).

FIGURE 3

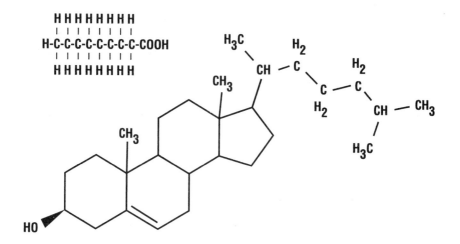

A saturated fat molecule (top left) and a cholesterol molecule (above).

As James Black warned over 200 years ago:

> A nice adaptation of conditions will make almost any hypothesis
> agree with the phenomena. This will please the imagination, but
> does not advance our knowledge.
>
> BLACK, J, *LECTURES OF THE ELEMENTS OF CHEMISTRY*, 1803

Unfortunately, this adaptation did not work. It is true that Ancel
Keys appeared to have proven the link between saturated-fat
consumption and heart disease, but, when it came to the major
interventional trials, confirmation proved elusive.

The MR-FIT trial in the USA was the most determined effort to
prove the case. This was a massive study in which over 350,000 men
at high risk of heart disease were recruited. In one set of participants
they cut cholesterol consumption by 42 per cent, saturated-fat
consumption by 28 per cent and total calories by 21 per cent. This
should have made a noticeable dent in heart-disease rates.

But nothing happened. The originators of the MR-FIT trials refer
to the results as 'disappointing' and say in their conclusions, 'The
overall results do not show a beneficial effect on coronary heart
disease or total mortality from this multifactor intervention.'

In fact, no clinical trial on reducing saturated-fat intake has
ever shown a reduction in heart disease. Some have shown the
exact opposite:

> As multiple intervention against risk factors for coronary heart
> disease in middle-aged men at only moderate risk seem to have
> failed to reduce both morbidity and mortality, such
> interventions become increasingly difficult to justify. This runs
> counter to the recommendations of many national and
> international advisory bodies which must now take the recent
> findings from Finland into consideration. Not to do so may be
> ethically unacceptable.
>
> PROFESSOR MICHAEL OLIVER, *BMJ*, 1991

This quote followed a disturbing trial on Finnish businessmen. In a 10-year follow-up to the original five-year trial, it was found that those men who continued to follow a low-saturated-fat diet were *twice* as likely to die of heart disease as those who didn't.

It is not even as if this was one negative to set against a whole series of positive trials. In 1998, Uffe Ravnskov looked at a broader selection of trials. 'The crucial test,' he decided, 'is the controlled, randomised trial. Eight such trials using diet as the only treatment have been performed, but neither the number of fatal or non-fatal heart attacks was reduced.' As Ravnskov makes clear, no trial has *ever* demonstrated benefits from reducing dietary saturated fat.

At this point, most people might think, it would be time to pull the plug. Far from it. In 1988, the surgeon general's office in the USA decided to silence the naysayers by putting together *the* definitive report proving a causal link. Eleven years later, the project was abandoned. In a letter circulated, it was stated that the office 'did not anticipate fully the magnitude of the additional external expertise and staff resources that would be needed'.

Bill Harlan, a member of the oversight committee and associate director of the Office of Disease Prevention at the National Institute of Health, says, 'The report was initiated with a preconceived opinion of the conclusions, but the science behind those opinions was not holding up. Clearly, the thoughts of yesterday were not going to serve us very well.'

The sound of a sinking cathedral filled the air with a great sucking, slurripy noise. But still no one let go. Instead, more buttresses were desperately thrown at a rapidly disappearing pile of rocks.

Variations on a theme emerged. It is not saturated fat per se that causes heart disease; it is the ratio of polyunsaturated to saturated fat that is critical. Or is it the consumption of monounsaturated fats, or a lack of omega-3 fatty acids, or an excess of omega-6? Take your pick. These, and a host of other add-on hypotheses, have their proponents. As of today, no one will – or can – tell you which type of fat, in what proportions, added to what type of antioxidant, vegetable, monounsaturated fat or omega-3 is the true culprit. Hugely complicated explanations are formulated, but they all fall apart under scrutiny.

This may all seem incredible, such has been the level of anti-fat propaganda, but it is true. With the exception of the Ancel Keys's unconvincing Seven Countries Study (he pre-selected the seven countries for his study), there is not one scrap of direct evidence.

But, of course, there are two parts to the cholesterol hypothesis. The diet part, and the raised cholesterol-level part. Leaving diet behind, surely it has been proven beyond doubt that a raised cholesterol level *is* the most important cause of heart disease...

CHOLESTEROL LEVELS AND OVERALL MORTALITY

Before looking at the connection between blood cholesterol levels and heart disease, I think it is worth highlighting a critically important – remarkably unheralded – fact: after the age of 50, the lower your cholesterol level, the lower your life expectancy.

Perhaps even more important than this is the fact that a falling cholesterol level sharply increases the risk of dying of anything, including heart disease. The dangers of a low cholesterol level were highlighted by a major long-term study of men living in Honolulu: 'Our data accord with previous findings of increased mortality in elderly people with low serum cholesterol, and show that long-term persistence of low cholesterol concentration actually increases the risk of death.'

The danger of a falling cholesterol level was first discovered (somewhat ironically) in the Framingham study: 'There is a direct association between falling cholesterol levels over the first 14 years [of the study] and mortality over the following 18 years.'

It seems almost unbelievable that warnings about the dangers of a high cholesterol level rain down every day, when the reality is that a *low* cholesterol level is much more dangerous than a high level. Given this, why would anyone want to lower the cholesterol level? On the face of it, it would make more sense to take cholesterol-raising drugs, especially after the age of 50.

CHOLESTEROL LEVELS AND HEART DISEASE

The reason why everyone is so keen to lower cholesterol levels is that supporters of the hypothesis have decreed the following:

A high level of cholesterol *causes* premature heart disease.

A low level of cholesterol is caused *by* an underlying disease.

It is the underlying disease that kills you, not the low cholesterol.

Ergo, if you lower the blood cholesterol level, you will reduce the risk of heart disease, and you will *not* increase the risk of dying of any other disease.

This could be true, but it is worth reviewing some of the evidence that linked raised cholesterol levels to heart disease in the first place. Let's begin with women.

Perhaps the largest single analysis of cholesterol levels and death from cardiovascular disease (and other diseases) was published in 1992. This review included over 100,000 women, aggregated from a number of different studies and countries.

To quote from the study: 'The pooled estimated risk for total cardiovascular death in women showed no trend across TC (total cholesterol) levels.' In short, for more than 50 per cent of the world's population – women – raised cholesterol is not a risk factor for heart disease.

Moving to men, it is true that under the age of 50, there does seem to be an association between raised cholesterol levels and heart disease. But, after the age of 50, when more than 90 per cent of heart attacks happen, the association disappears.

In addition, those populations in the world with the highest rates of heart disease in younger men – including emigrant Asian Indians, Eastern Europeans, Native Americans and Australian Aboriginals – tend to have significantly lower cholesterol levels than the surrounding populations/countries.

Perhaps the single most directly contradictory fact is that, in young Japanese men, the average cholesterol level has risen over the last 20

FIGURE 4

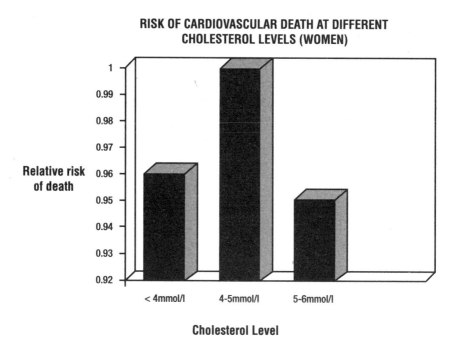

RISK OF CARDIOVASCULAR DEATH AT DIFFERENT
CHOLESTEROL LEVELS (WOMEN)

Risk of cardiovascular death at different cholesterol levels (women).

years, yet the rate of heart disease has fallen. But, as with many facts in this area, if they don't fit the cholesterol hypothesis, they are dismissed.

LOWERING CHOLESTEROL LEVELS WITH DRUGS

Surely, despite everything written up to this point, all previous arguments are refuted by the knowledge that lowering cholesterol levels with statins protects against heart disease. As all good scientists know, that 'reversibility of effect' provides the most powerful supportive evidence for a hypothesis.

However, there is a flip side to this argument: how can lowering cholesterol levels prevent heart disease in people who do *not* have a high level? The most often quoted clinical trial in the last few years is the UK-based Heart Protection Study (HPS) – a veritable triumph for statins, demonstrating protection in almost every group studied.

What is most intriguing, however, is that protection was apparent if the starting cholesterol level was high, average or low. How can this be explained?

At this point we enter *Alice in Wonderland* territory. A rational person would accept that a *normal* cholesterol level cannot be a risk factor for heart disease (or anything else for that matter). Therefore, people with normal cholesterol levels can gain no benefit from having their levels lowered.

Ergo, if statins *do* protect those with normal, or low, cholesterol levels – which they clearly do – they must be doing this through some other mechanism or action, unrelated to cholesterol lowering.

In fact, there is a growing body of evidence to support the idea that statins have a whole series of different protective actions. But accepting that statins work in another way would demolish the final buttress keeping the cholesterol hypothesis afloat. And so the latest argument is that no one in modern society has a normal cholesterol level. An article in the *Journal of the American College of Cardiology* best sums up this line of thinking. Under the heading 'Why average is not normal', O'Keefe, the lead author, makes the claim that 'Atherosclerosis is endemic in our population, in part because the average LDL ['bad' cholesterol – of which more later] level is approximately twice the normal physiologic level'. In short, according to O'Keefe, our cholesterol level should be about 2.5 mmol/l, not 5.2 mmol/l.

This argument, if true, does neatly demolish the question of how people with normal, or low, cholesterol levels can be protected against heart disease. O'Keefe and others would argue that we *all* have a high cholesterol level. Everyone is ill, and all shall have statins.

One regularly quoted fact, which seems superficially supportive of O'Keefe's hypothesis, is that peasant farmers in China have very low cholesterol levels and a very low rate of heart disease (although their average cholesterol levels are actually about four, not two and a half). But, when you study the figures with more care, they reveal something else. As usual, those with low cholesterol levels have by far the highest mortality rates – liver failure and liver cancer are common causes of death. However, there is a simple explanation for this association: many Chinese peasant farmers have chronic hepatitis which creates low cholesterol levels, and also leads to liver failure and liver cancer, which is why people with low cholesterol levels die young.

Does this mean that a low cholesterol level protects against heart disease? No, what the Chinese data tell us is that those with higher cholesterol levels are *not* chronic hepatitis carriers, so they live longer and have more chance of developing heart disease in old age. On the other hand, those with low cholesterol levels cannot die of heart disease, because they are already dead.

Without chasing too many mad arguments around, the simple fact is that everyone in the West does *not* have a raised cholesterol level. Repeated studies have shown that a perfectly normal, or healthy, cholesterol level lies between about four and six, and lowering it cannot protect against heart disease, otherwise we will have introduced a new concept into medical science: normal is unhealthy and must be treated.

People are grasping at straws in their attempt to explain why statins protect against heart disease in those with normal cholesterol levels, and in women and the elderly where a raised cholesterol level is not even a risk factor. The only possible explanation for the results of the statin trials is that statins do *not* work by lowering cholesterol levels.

THE CHOLESTEROL HYPOTHESIS IS A COMPLICATED MESS

The cholesterol hypothesis has always exuded the siren song of simplicity. However, once you start to examine it in any detail, the simplicity rapidly mutates into complexity. Even at the very start, people should have known that cholesterol in the diet was never capable of appearing, unchanged, in the bloodstream. Cholesterol is not soluble in water (thus blood) which means that, after absorption, cells lining the gut pack cholesterol into a small protein/lipid sphere, known as a lipoprotein, before releasing it into the bloodstream.

Thus, you do not have any cholesterol floating about in the blood; it is all contained within lipoproteins. You do not actually have a cholesterol level. Instead, you have a level of different lipoproteins with the low-density lipoprotein (LDL) or 'bad' cholesterol being the so-called dangerous one.

Next question: what raises the LDL level? Eating too much fat, or cholesterol? The first problem here is that the cells lining the gut do not make, or release, LDL – they make other forms of lipoprotein. So, no matter what you eat, it can have no direct effect on LDL levels.

So where does LDL come from? LDL is, effectively, the shrunken form of a very low-density lipoprotein (VLDL). VLDLs are made in the liver and used to transport fat, and cholesterol, from the liver to other cells around the body. As VLDLs lose fat they shrink, transforming into LDL. Therefore, in order to find out what makes LDL levels rise, we must surely find out, first, what makes VLDL levels go up; and what makes VLDL levels go up, primarily, is eating excess carbohydrates. What makes them go down is eating fat!

Recognising this, and a host of other problems, the supporters of the cholesterol hypothesis have turned and turned. As of today (and this will certainly change), the original – dietary – cholesterol hypothesis has become the following: if you eat too much saturated fat, the body will reduce the number of LDL receptors (things that remove LDL from the bloodstream), forcing the LDL up. A more tenuous, and unproven, link could hardly be imagined, but that is what is left of the originally super-simple cholesterol hypothesis – the diet part, anyway.

But the difficulties of trying to establish a dietary link to heart disease actually pale into insignificance when you start trying to work out how the raised LDL level itself may cause heart disease.

If it were simply a case of excess LDL seeping through the artery wall when the level gets too high, then why doesn't this happen in all artery walls, everywhere? If I lie too long in the sun, I expect to get sunburned on every bit of skin exposed. I do not expect to get discrete patches of sunburn. Yet we do see little 'patches' of atherosclerosis. Some people who die of heart disease are found to have perfectly clean arteries, apart from a single killer plaque. So why did the LDL seep through at only one place? What protected the rest of the arterial system?

And why do veins never develop atherosclerotic plaques? They are exposed to exactly the same LDL level as the arteries. They are thinner than arteries, but their general structure is identical. I should add that, if you use a vein as a coronary artery bypass graft (effectively turning it into an artery), it will develop atherosclerosis.

These questions are just the beginning. In an attempt to answer some of them, the cholesterol hypothesis has turned itself into the following, complicated mess. LDL, when it is oxidised, travels through the lining of the artery wall (endothelium) into the middle part of the artery. (*How oxidised LDL passes straight through an endothelial cell into the artery wall behind is unexplained.*) In this oxidised state it attracts white blood cells from the bloodstream They, in turn, migrate into the artery wall and start to 'digest' the oxidised LDL in order to remove it. (*This bit is plausible.*) However, white blood cells, once they have started to digest oxidised LDL, cannot stop. They get bigger and bigger until they burst. This, in turn, attracts more white blood cells to the area, which then also burst. (*White blood cells that just burst? This makes absolutely no sense whatsoever. Why on earth would the body develop a scavenger system that automatically self-destructs?*) The burst white blood cells, in turn, release substances that trigger a whole cascade of inflammatory reactions in the arterial wall. After a period of time you have a mass of dead white blood cells, cholesterol, oxidised LDL remnants, and a whole series of other inflammatory agents all focused in one area, trapped in the artery wall. (*Well, this is what is found in a plaque, among many other things.*)

Anyway, that is allegedly how a plaque starts and grows. I have kept that explanation as simple as humanly possible, but it seems absurdly unlikely. Oxidised LDL – what happened to normal LDL?

Well, there's no way anyone can see of getting that through an arterial wall. Exploding white blood cells – another buttress?

In truth, the current ideas on plaque formation that are used to keep the cholesterol hypothesis afloat are complex nonsense. But the entire area is now protected by a ring-fence of scientific jargon which frightens off all but the most dedicated truth-seeker. To those who have studied the hypothesis with a critical eye, it seems unbelievable that it can possibly still be standing. Dr George Mann pronounced it dead in an editorial in the *New England Journal of Medicine* in 1977, referring to it as the 'greatest scam in the history of medicine'. Yet this hypothesis has never had more followers than today. Time, I think, that it was consigned to the dustbin of history. It is neither simple, direct nor understandable; the only certain thing about it is that it is wrong.

Chapter Eighteen

GENETICALLY MODIFIED ORGANISMS

BY SIR PETER LACHMANN

The Myth: **Genetically modified foods are harmful to human health.**

The Fact: **The reported health benefits of genetically modified foods are substantial, the hazards non-existent.**

INTRODUCTION

By contrast with BSE, where there were serious problems and risks to human as well as animal health that required substantial scientific work to evaluate and control, the public furore about health hazards of genetically modified foods rests on no reliable evidence base and falls little short of mass hysteria. It is a story whose interest lies not in its science reality but in the way that the mishandled commercial introduction of two particular GM products allowed an alliance of pressure groups and campaigning media, with a witches' brew of anti-science agendas, to alarm the public and bring about a situation that is both farcical and alarming. In this short summary, the scientific background of genetic-modification technology and its application to food crops are discussed, along with the question of what risks, if any, it may pose to both human and animal health.

THE SCIENTIFIC BACKGROUND

The 'molecular biological revolution' began with the observation in 1928 by British bacteriologist Fred Griffith that injecting mice with a mixture of heat-killed, virulent pneumococci and living, non-virulent pneumococci killed the mice, from which virulent living organisms could then be recovered. This first observation of genetic modification – the gene for virulence having been picked up by the living bacteria from the dead ones – was a *discovery* not an *invention*. It is a natural process that bacteria use all the time. Avery and his colleagues in New York showed in 1943 – to everyone's great surprise – that it was DNA that was responsible for producing this transformation, thereby showing that DNA was the genetic material.

In 1953 Watson and Crick published their double-helix structure for DNA from which the mechanism of DNA replication was readily deduced and led on to the sequencing of DNA and eventually of whole genomes. However, it was not until the 1970s that a number of new discoveries – in apparently unrelated fields – came together to allow the manipulation of genes. (This is often called 'recombinant DNA technology' or 'genetic engineering'.) These were the discovery of: bacterial plasmids – the DNA-containing particles that transfer genetic material (for example, genes coding for antibiotic resistance) between bacteria; 'restriction endonucleases', bacterial enzymes that clip DNA with sequence specificity; and 'reverse transcriptase', a viral enzyme that copies RNA back into DNA, which is necessary for the replication of some viruses. By making use of these three discoveries it became possible to clone and to manipulate genes. At first the technology was quite difficult and time-consuming, but technical advances, notably a chemical way of reproducing DNA by the 'polymerase chain reaction' in the early 1980s, allowed its widespread use in biology and medicine.

Many applications of genetic engineering in medicine are well established and not at all controversial. These include the recombinant protein vaccine against Hepatitis B, which has been hugely successful in reducing the incidence of this important disease and in preventing many cases of liver cancer. Because the earlier plasma-derived vaccine always carried the danger of contamination with unknown viruses, the recombinant vaccine is much to be preferred both on the grounds of safety and efficacy. Another example is the use of recombinant growth hormone to treat children with dwarfism. Since the growth hormone extracted from human pituitary glands was able to transmit Creutzfeld Jacob Disease, the new recombinant product was very welcome.

The first application of genetic engineering to food was 'vegetarian cheese'. Strict vegetarians object to eating hard cheese where the milk is first curdled with rennet, an enzyme derived from calves' stomachs which involves killing the calf. To avoid using rennet, cheese manufacturers started using chymase, an enzyme made from genetically engineered yeast instead. This was accepted without any opposition. The first genetically modified food plant was the 'FlavrSavr' tomato, which has a genetic modification (an antisense polygalacturonase gene) to delay softening. It was introduced to the market rather cautiously and was also accepted without obvious controversy.

The present furore has its origins in the introduction of two genetically modified commodity crops by Monsanto, and particularly by the unwise mixing of the GM products with the harvests from unmodified crops so that the consumers could not know whether the product contained genetically modified material. The two introduced genes (or transgenes) involved were:

1. A gene that makes a plant resistant to the herbicide glyphosphate, which can then be used to kill the weeds in the crop. Oil seed rape and soya were modified in this way.
2. The *Bacillus thuringiensis* toxin, which confers resistance to stem-boring insects. (This toxin is used in organic agriculture when applied as a spray of whole bacteria.) Maize was modified in this way.

These introductions were not well received! A coalition of those opposed to corporate agriculture and to big business as a whole joined with those opposed to science as a whole and those worried particularly about genetics and 'playing God'; others, not least in the media, saw an opportunity for publicity and gain; and a group of maverick scientists – now inevitably involved in any media controversy about science – instituted a campaign to persuade the public that GMOs were a conspiracy against poor farmers, a fraud on the gullibility of those farmers who grow them, an intrinsic evil and a hazard to human health and the environment.

In the United Kingdom, the GMO situation was particularly inflamed by the affair of Dr Pusztai and the GM potatoes. Dr Pusztai worked at the Rowett Institute in Aberdeen, which took part in a research project to study whether introducing lectins (plant proteins that naturally protect against insects) into other plants could improve their resistance to insects. Purely for this research (and with no intention of introducing them as a commercial product), potatoes were made transgenic for snowdrop lectin and these transgenic potatoes were tested in a variety of ways. Dr Pusztai, who had worked on lectins as anti-cancer agents, participated in experiments involving feeding transgenic potatoes to rats. These experiments had major problems. The worst was that only one line of congenic potato had been made and this had not been bred further to construct 'congenic' lines of potato that were identical, other than for the presence of the transgene. The single transgenic potato line was compared with ordinary potatoes; many differences, unrelated to the transgene, will have been present between the two. The only meaningful way, short of breeding congenics, of conducting these experiments would have been to make many lines of transgenic potatoes and compare them with many lines of potatoes that had not been transfected. This was not done and caused Dr Gatehouse, who had done the genetic manipulation of the potatoes, subsequently to dissociate himself from the work. However, the first that the wider world heard of any of this was when Dr Pusztai appeared on a *World in Action* TV programme in August 1998 and told the audience that genetically modified potatoes affected organ weights in rats and damaged their immune system. He put the relevant data on to the Internet, and at that time a journalist invited me to take a look at them. It was clear, even without knowing that the potato lines were not congenic, that the experiments could have been improved upon, showed only small and not clearly interpretable effects and used a faulty statistical analysis. In view of the public interest, the Royal Society issued a statement prepared by a working party. It concluded that 'the work was flawed in many aspects of design, execution and analysis and that no conclusion should be drawn from it'. This statement raised the ire of Richard Horton, the editor of *The Lancet*, who claimed it to be 'breathtaking impertinence' on behalf of the Royal Society to get involved. What is and what is not impertinence is clearly very much in the eye of the beholder.

In 1999, *The Lancet* poured more petrol on the flames by publishing a paper by Ewen and Pusztai based on the same experiments (the only ones that had been done at the Rowett) but presenting different results from those that had been put on the Internet and criticised. They now claimed that there was a reduction in gut mucosal thickness and a small increase in the number of intraepithelial lymphocytes. This paper was also deeply flawed on the grounds of selection of data, the absence of a proper control group and, again, faulty statistics. In this case, the statistics had been improved upon by *The Lancet* statistician who had not been informed these were data 'dredged' from the earlier experiments.

For unknown reasons, and from a source that has never been revealed, corrected author proofs of this paper were widely circulated before it was published. This caused there to be considerable protest even before the paper appeared. Most significantly, John Gatehouse wrote to Richard Horton explaining where the work was faulty and disassociating himself from it. Under the guidelines of the Committee on Publication Ethics (of which Richard Horton was a member), this made the paper unpublishable since all significant contributors to work must give their consent to its publication. This letter is said to have reached *The Lancet* after it had gone to press, but there can be no excuse for its not subsequently being published and the paper withdrawn. Horton declined to do this on the grounds that, since the letter had appeared on John Gatehouse's website, it could not be published in *The Lancet*.

I telephoned Richard Horton before publication to tell him that I regarded publishing such a flawed paper as wrong, and we had a somewhat acrimonious conversation. To my considerable surprise, the contents of our conversation subsequently appeared in an article on the front page of the *Guardian*, with the addition of the entirely untrue allegation that I had threatened Richard Horton that his position would be in peril if he published the paper. I can only imagine that someone felt that something of this nature was required to make the story sufficiently newsworthy, and it certainly received a great deal of attention on the anti-GM websites, if not elsewhere.

This episode demonstrates the extent to which the GM-food debate had abandoned the arena of scientific discourse for that of a media circus. The role of *The Lancet* in this matter – as in the later affair of Dr Wakefield and the MMR vaccine – has hardly enhanced its reputation among the medical and scientific community. Not unexpectedly, the publication was used by anti-GMO campaigners as a vindication of their stance, although it was almost universally repudiated by scientific commentators. Dr Pusztai, now retired, has established himself as a victim of scientific oppression and as a scientific hero for the anti-GMO lobby – a role that he clearly enjoys (see www.freenetpages.co.uk/hp/a.pusztai).

DO GMOS PRESENT HEALTH RISKS?

Dr Pusztai's potatoes apart, are there any reasons to be concerned about the health effects of genetic modification of food? It is essential here to distinguish the effects of genetic modification as a procedure from the effects of any particular introduced transgene. As far as the procedure itself is concerned, there is absolutely no reason to suppose that it is harmful to human health. The only suggestion that one particular method of introducing transgenes could be harmful comes from Mai-Wan Ho and her colleagues who have suggested that the use of a cauliflower mosaic virus promoter can lead to recombination with viruses such as Hepatitis B or HIV to create lethal super-viruses. There is, however, not a scrap of evidence for any such thing. Viruses can recombine only when replicating their genomes inside cells, a situation where the possibility of encountering any CMV promoter from food is exceedingly remote. Plant promoters in general do not interact with animal viruses; if they did, we would have known about it, since we eat large quantities of CMV in our normal diet. This hazard would appear to be a fantasy.

The possible toxic effects of introducing a new transgene, either as a result of the properties of the transgene itself or because of secondary effects on the plant, need to be tested, just as all new foodstuffs need to be tested for toxicity and allergenicity. The two major GMOs on the market at the moment, discussed above, have been eaten for many years by very large numbers of people in the United States and in China, and there is really not even any anecdotal suggestion that they may do any damage. Indeed, making maize resistant to stem-boring insects reduces the incidence of secondary fungal infection and there is experimental evidence that one mycotoxin, fumonisin, which is considered unsafe for horses and pigs, shows a 90 per cent reduction in these cereals compared to the non-transgenic types. The same seems to be true of aflatoxin which, in patients carrying Hepatitis B or Hepatitis C viruses, is an important cause of liver cancer. For this particular transgene, therefore, the only documented health effects are favourable.

WHAT, THEN, ARE THE ANTI-GM ARGUMENTS?

1. GMOs in reality give no advantage to the farmer and do not have the beneficial properties claimed for them, for example reducing insecticide use and giving better yields. This is a curious argument for a lobby group to employ since, if true, there is really nothing to lobby about.

Farmers are unlikely to grow crops which are of no benefit to them.

2. GM foods are a conspiracy against the public by large agrochemical companies that wish to dominate world agriculture, damage the livelihood of poor farmers and expose the unsuspecting consumer as well as the environment to unknown risks. Conspiracy theories are notoriously difficult to refute as the counter-arguments are then represented as an example of further conspiracies!

The anti-GMO campaign has overtones of moral fanaticism – GMOs are not just undesirable, they are actually evil – which it shares with the campaigns against genetic intervention in human reproduction. However, while the latter have some religious basis, the major religious groups, including the Vatican, have declined to endorse the anti-GMO campaign. There is also no doubt that the anti-GM groups have access to considerable sources of finance. One of the British websites devoted entirely to this subject is GMWatch (www.gmwatch.org) which publishes profiles of all the many organisations and individuals that they regard as part of the conspiracy to force-feed the public with GMOs. For this they acknowledge financial support from a foundation known as the JMG Foundation. This is described on the Internet (www.undueinfluence.com/jmg_foundation.htm) as an 'Anti-corporate, anti-capitalist foundation created with part of the fortune of the late billionaire, Sir James Michael Goldsmith. It funds aggressive campaign to destroy biotech crop production worldwide, member of International Forum on Globalization and Funders Network on Trade and Globalization'. Its only reported trustee is Edward Goldsmith, the brother of the late Sir James. This might appear an ironic source of funds for such a purpose.

THE FUTURE OF GMOS

There is no question that the selective modification of food plants that is possible using techniques of genetic modification is both more precise and more controllable than conventional plant breeding, and it will also be much quicker. Once the media furore has abated or, more probably, fixed its attention on some different topic, genetic modification of food plants will surely become an entirely routine, uncontroversial and everyday facet of plant breeding.

It carries huge potential. The present products are very much the 'horseless carriage' phase of its development, and in the middle future and beyond there are much more important and significant gains to be achieved. The improvement of nutritional quality of foods, for example, by modifying protein and fatty-acid composition is certainly possible, and one improved food – 'golden rice', which makes beta-carotene – is already available. The elimination of known allergens and toxic compounds is also possible, as are food-based vaccines. One agricultural aim is to breed more salt-tolerant crops and thereby restore saline-polluted land to agricultural use. This would carry great economic benefits to many poor countries. There is the prospect of engineering cereals to fix nitrogen from the air (as legumes do), thereby reducing the use of nitrogenous fertilisers. This is not going to be easy, since this process uses many genes, but it is potentially achievable. The most ambitious project is to increase the efficiency of photosynthesis. The late Lord Porter pointed out that, if one could increase the efficiency of photosynthesis from around 1 per cent to around 5 per cent, one could not only feed all the world from agriculture but also provide all its energy needs. It is not clear that this is possible, but it would be a great triumph.

The future is bright enough, but getting there will need both courage and perseverance.

Chapter Nineteen

THE MMR STORY

BY MICHAEL FITZPATRICK

The Myth: **The MMR vaccine causes autism in children.**

The Fact: **There is no evidence to suggest that this is the case.**

The announcement of a new 'five in one' immunisation for babies
in August 2004 might have been expected to receive popular
approval. The new combination jab includes the familiar tetanus and
diphtheria vaccines, safer and more effective vaccines against
whooping cough and polio, as well as providing additional
protection against meningitis caused by *Haemophilus influenzae*
type B. Furthermore, it does not contain the mercury-based
preservative thiomersal, which has been blamed by some
campaigners (without scientific confirmation) for causing
neurodevelopmental disorders in children.

Yet, far from being a cause for celebration, the new vaccine
provoked another anti-immunisation media panic. The writer
Carmen Reid declared that she was 'furious' with the government
and warned that 'anybody coming near my children with a new
improved vaccination can take a running jump'. Reid was almost
apoplectic with rage over the introduction of a new vaccine

offering a wider range of protection with lower risks of adverse reactions. Why?

It is not easy to explain the intensity of the anger of anti-vaccine campaigners. The ostensible focus of their fury is an implied conspiracy among the government, the drug companies and the doctors to conceal the grievous dangers that they believe may result from vaccines. So let's look first at concerns about their possible adverse effects, particularly the alleged link with autism that has provoked so much parental anxiety. We can then turn to examine what lies behind popular anxieties about vaccines.

THE MMR DEBACLE

In the notorious February 1998 *Lancet* paper that launched the MMR scare, Dr Andrew Wakefield and colleagues wrote that 'we did not prove a link between MMR vaccine and this syndrome ('autistic enterocolitis')'. Nor have they proved it in the seven years since.

In February 2004, following revelations that Dr Wakefield had failed to declare a conflict of interest arising from his acceptance of £10,000 in legal-aid funding from the anti-MMR litigation, 10 of his co-authors issued a 'partial retraction' of the paper. This withdrew claims of a link between MMR and autism, but insisted that the identification of a distinctive form of inflammatory bowel disease in children with autism remained valid. For many critics, the possible bias in the selection of the dozen cases for the *Lancet* study meant that it was also impossible to have any confidence in the concept of 'autistic enterocolitis'. Many of the parents were referred to Dr Wakefield's clinic at the Royal Free Hospital in north London following their earlier exposure to the anti-MMR campaign and to Dr Wakefield's theories of a link between measles (or measles vaccination) and inflammatory bowel disease.

The four links in the proposed chain of causality connecting MMR to autism are speculative – none has been substantiated. They are:

1. 'MMR immunisation leads to chronic measles infection (and

immune dysfunction).' Although it is well known that MMR may cause minor adverse reactions, it has never been shown to cause measles. Nor has the combination of live (attenuated) viruses in MMR been shown to suppress or otherwise damage the infant immune system.

2. 'Measles causes "autistic enterocolitis".' Apart from the discredited 1998 *Lancet* paper and other publications by the same authors, no properly validated research has confirmed the existence of this condition. Claims that studies by Dublin virologist John O'Leary have confirmed an MMR-autism link, mediated by measles-related bowel inflammation, have been repudiated by Professor O'Leary himself.

3. 'A leaky bowel allows toxic opiod peptides to enter the blood stream.' Children with autism are not particularly prone to have leaky bowels and opiod peptides are not toxic (they are produced naturally in the body during acupuncture, exposure to sunlight and sexual activity).

4. '"Opioid excess" in the brain causes autism.' Only based on the assumption that autistic children behave like laboratory animals on opiates and is entirely speculative.

The Medical Research Council considered this proposed causal sequence 'biologically implausible'.

Because MMR is given after 12 months and the features of autism often become apparent at around 18 months, it is not surprising that, in cases where behavioural regression appeared soon after vaccination, some parents have blamed the vaccine. However, exhaustive epidemiological researches, conducted with different methods in different countries, have failed to confirm any causal relationship.

In response to the failure of virological and epidemiological research to confirm the MMR–autism hypothesis, its supporters have shifted ground. In the cases reported in the *Lancet*, autistic features appeared – on average – within six days of the MMR jab (though an auto-immune process causing bowel inflammation would require several weeks).

One of the most popular claims of the anti-MMR campaign is that MMR is to blame for an 'epidemic of autism'. Since studies have failed to reveal any link between the introduction of MMR and the rise in diagnoses of autism, campaigners now claim that MMR is to blame for only a small subset of autism cases, one too small to measure by epidemiological methods.

As the alleged link between the MMR vaccine and autism has been discredited, anti-immunisation campaigners in Britain have shifted their attention to vaccines containing the mercury-based preservative thiomersal. This has long been the main focus of campaigners in the USA. Mercury is potentially toxic to the central nervous system and particularly to the developing infant brain, but the total exposure to mercury resulting from the vaccines traditionally administered in the UK over the first six months of life is well below the WHO recommended safety threshold (which itself incorporates a tenfold safety factor). Babies are likely to receive higher doses of mercury if their mothers consume fish such as shark, marlin and swordfish which are known to contain relatively high levels of mercury.

Campaigners claim that the symptoms of mercury toxicity are similar to those of autism. On closer inspection, the clinical features of both conditions are quite distinct. Mercury poisoning causes a staggering gait, slurring speech, visual-field disturbances and peripheral neuropathy. In mild cases, it produces a non-specific anxiety and depression; in more severe cases, a toxic psychosis may result. None of these features is characteristic of autism.

There have been a number of well-recognised epidemics of mercury poisoning. The most notorious, known as 'pink disease', resulted from the widespread use of proprietary teething powders containing mercury during the first half of the twentieth century. Infants with this condition displayed painful, pink and peeling hands and feet. Though pink disease caused more than 100 deaths a year in Britain into the 1940s, survivors have never been reported as displaying disorders such as autism.

Vaccines containing mercury have been in use for more than 60 years, during which time they have saved countless lives and prevented numerous cases of disability, without causing any more serious problem than an occasional allergic reaction. In February 2003, the UK Committee on Safety of Medicines reviewed two studies of mercury containing vaccines, involving more than 100,000 children, and found no association with autism. In February 2004, in response to continuing claims of links between vaccines and autism, the US Institute of Medicine reviewed the evidence and rejected a causal relationship between both mercury-containing vaccines and MMR and autism. It upheld the current child-immunisation schedule.

The removal of thiomersal-containing vaccines from the child programme has not succeeded in quelling anxieties. While some argued that this merely vindicated earlier claims about the dangers of mercury, others discovered new dangers. According to Carmen Reid's denunciation of the 'five-in-one' vaccine, 'instead of mercury, the new vaccination contains aluminium and formaldehyde, both known neurological toxins, held by some [unidentified experts] to be responsible for autism'. In fact, aluminium is present in some proprietary medicines that are available in pharmacies and it has never caused any toxicity, although exposure to high concentrations of aluminium in the drinking water in Camelford caused some skin irritation.

COMBINATION

A recurrent theme in parental concerns about MMR, one that has been carried over into the response to the new 'five-in-one' jab, is that the combination of vaccines is damaging to the infantile immune system. However, although children receive more vaccines today than in the past, the higher quality of the vaccines means that the number of antigens they receive has declined. For example, the old smallpox vaccine, which was used until smallpox was eradicated in the 1970s, contained 200 proteins. Now the 11 vaccines routinely administered in the USA contain fewer than 130 proteins (and more than half of these are in the chickenpox vaccine that has yet to be introduced in Britain).

According to US vaccine specialist Paul Offit and colleagues, the infant immune system has the theoretical capacity to respond to 'about 10,000 vaccines at any one time'. Put another way, they reckon that, if all 11 vaccines were given at the same time, 'then about 0.1 per cent of the immune system would be "used up"'. They insist that 'young infants have an enormous capacity to respond to multiple vaccines, as well as to the many other challenges present in the environment'.

A study in Britain looked specifically at the impact of the MMR combination on the immune system. The authors hypothesised that 'if MMR vaccine does induce clinically significant immunosuppression, susceptibility to infection should be increased in the post-vaccination period'. They found that there was no increased risk of hospitalisation with infections such as pneumonia within three months of vaccination; indeed, there was a slight protective effect.

DEFAULTERS AND RESISTERS

Following its introduction in the UK in 1988, uptake of MMR rose steadily to reach a peak of 92 per cent in 1995. It began to fall in 1997 – before the publication of Dr Wakefield's *Lancet* paper in 1998, after which it fell further. The decline accelerated in the early 2000s as the anti-MMR campaign gathered momentum. By 2003, uptake had fallen to 80 per cent nationally, and 70 per cent in London. Who were the people who were choosing not to give their babies the triple vaccine?

Passive defaulters, whose children were not being immunised, were characteristically low-income families experiencing various forms of deprivation and social exclusion. Their failure to have their children immunised was partly attributed to 'parental reluctance' and partly to 'professional apathy', the poor provision of primary care and child-health services, notably in inner-city areas.

Active resisters to immunisation were middle-class, well-educated parents who had chosen not to have their children immunised. These parents were concerned about the risks of adverse consequences of immunisation, which they felt had been played down in the official information. They often expressed sceptical views towards 'biomedicine' and an openness to alternatives, particularly homeopathy. They were suspicious of the apparent convergence of interests among the medical profession, the government and the vaccine manufacturers.

It was the expansion of the numbers of active resisters that reduced uptake of MMR to levels that made outbreaks of measles (and mumps and rubella) a serious possibility, especially in London. There was a convergence between radical ecological and traditional conservative values in environmentalist and consumerist campaigns. Anti-immunisation sentiment united elements from diverse and often conflicting political traditions.

THE RAGE OF SUBURBIA

The angry press response to the introduction of the new 'five-in-one' vaccine cannot be explained solely as a response to changes in the child-immunisation schedule. It can only be understood as an expression of the wider animosities of sections of the middle classes. A closer look at some of the targets of this outrage – the government, the drug companies and science itself – may shed some light on what is bothering the citizens of middle England.

The invasion and occupation of Iraq and the proposed ban on fox-hunting have provoked the biggest mass mobilisations against the government in Britain over the past decade. For some commentators, the new protest movements – involving many middle-aged, middle-class demonstrators – marked a welcome return to mass participation in politics. Yet the slogans arising from these protests reflected a sense of disengagement rather than any aspiration, let alone expectation, that the protestors might achieve their objectives. Condemnations of the prime minister for 'lying' or for 'not listening' to the concerns of the people expressed both a sense of rage and a feeling of powerlessness. 'They lied to us' was the childlike mantra that ran from the scandal over the spread of mad cow disease to humans, to the claim that Iraq's Saddam Hussein possessed 'weapons of mass destruction' as a pretext for war, to allegations of a cover-up over the risks of the MMR vaccine.

Another target that has attracted growing middle-class hostility is big business. Self-indulgent and backward-looking, the anti-capitalists of the 1990s tilted at windmills in the form of McDonalds and Starbucks. Yet such anti-corporate themes are no longer merely the preserve of left-wing weeklies, but can be found in comments on pharmaceutical companies and food manufacturers, as well as oil and tobacco companies, across the mass media and in academic publications, not least in medical journals. Like anti-government feeling, anti-corporate sentiment brings together elements of diverse political traditions. It incorporates the suspicion of the small businessman for the big corporation, the prejudice of the Little Englander against global – especially American, even European – capitalism.

A third factor in rising middle-class discontent is a growing scepticism about science, which is often combined with fears about environmental threats to health. Attitudes towards science and technology are characterised by a high degree of ambivalence. On the one hand, people embrace the iPod and other manifestations of technological advance with enthusiasm. On the other, they are fearful of the (speculative) risks of GM foods or advances in genetics and reproductive technology.

Visitors to Britain from overseas are bemused by the intensity of public controversy over issues of immunisation. In most other countries, immunisation is widely regarded as an important aspect of public-health policy and is generally uncontroversial – as it was in Britain up to the 1990s. Although in most countries there are small groups which reject immunisation on religious or ideological grounds, they have negligible influence on overall levels of vaccine uptake. A peculiar combination of factors in Britain in the late 1990s allowed the MMR scare to take off, putting the mass childhood-immunisation campaign as a whole in jeopardy.

The emergence of a maverick scientist – Dr Andrew Wakefield – was a key factor. Dr Wakefield's success in winning the support of a lawyer pursuing a class action on behalf of a substantial group of parents of autistic children who came to believe strongly in the MMR–autism theory gave the campaign legal-aid funding (up to a total of £15 million) and a strong base of support. Uncritical journalists who promoted Dr Wakefield's theory and his image as a champion of families affected by autism (and as victim of official persecution) provided vital publicity. The feeble and defensive response of the medical establishment, with a few distinguished but beleaguered exceptions, allowed the campaign to gather momentum.

Given the high level of free-floating anxieties and animosities we have identified among the British middle classes, the MMR scare found an immediate resonance, parents could refuse to have their children immunised or opt for separate vaccines. This assertion of parental rights had the effect of exposing their children to an increased risk of potentially serious infectious diseases. If significant outbreaks of measles occur – which now seems likely, particularly in London – the consequences of this misdirected parental rage could be tragic.

Chapter Twenty

SUN AND THE SKIN: A VIOLATION OF TRUTH

BY SAM SHUSTER

The Myth: Too much exposure to sunlight ages the skin and causes dangerous skin cancer.

The Fact: Exposure to sunlight has important health benefits and the cancers it has been proved to cause are functionally benign.

Anyone who has got this far in the book will have realised that there are so many medical perils lurking about that the only sure way to avoid them is death. This chapter is dedicated to those who would prefer to live.

Mankind and the sun have successfully maintained their unequal partnership for some considerable time. We owe our existence to it, and Darwinian genetic and social evolution long ago taught us how to cope with the quiddities of that existence and turn them to our advantage. For example, our bodies have developed the ability to use the sun for the production of the vitamin D that is essential for our bones and certain immune functions which it understands better than we do. Fortunately, that ability is passed on by the safe hand of genetic evolution, which is not subject to the vagaries of its social counterpart. For example, we have to learn not to look at the sun and how to avoid being burned by overexposure.

In the past, the lesson of such real experience was passed on socially; now unfortunately, our attitude to sun and ultraviolet (UV) light is subject to much perverse and dubious technical 'advice' which society has passively accepted without questioning its provenance. Whatever the subject, there is always a guru: for example there must be experts on the best way to tie shoelaces. To test this assertion I asked Google, and found 16,500 sites purporting to give the best way to tie shoelaces – and over half of a test sample gave the details! The problem is that there are now so many gurus on the dangers of sunshine that their shadow is obliterating the sun and our long-learned understanding of how to live with it.

We are told that we must severely limit our exposure to the sun and suntan lamps. If we must take a holiday where there is an opportunity to savour the delights of sunshine, we should avoid it as much as possible. The middle of the day should be considered dead time to be spent in the shade reading improving books. Leaflets in the doctor's surgery tell us we should wear wide-brimmed hats, long-sleeved shirts or blouses, and cover our legs. And we must not forget to cover ourselves with expensive, properly ranked, protective creams and lotions. As for the children, on the few precious occasions when the clouds of a British summer evaporate, we must not allow them out of doors before slapping on sticky sunscreens and bullying them into sweaty hats and clothes made with high sun-protective fabrics.

The reasons given for this punitive catalogue of dos and don'ts is that sun exposure ages the skin and causes cancer. Yet most things we do have risks: what matters is the consequence of that risk, and that depends upon the frequency and duration of exposure. Both have been grossly exaggerated for UV and its effect on the skin.

The rejuvenation of ageing skin is a money-spinner. There is no doubt whatsoever that exposure to UV radiation, particularly UVB (the shorter wavelength that causes sunburn but doesn't travel through window glass), gives skin a weather-beaten look, as does smoking. How long this takes and how severe it is depends on the dose of sun (or smoking) and your genetically determined response to it. The causal damage is to skin collagen, but this is only partly understood. We know that UV promotes molecular cross-links between collagen fibres, making them less elastic, but we do not really know the consequences of this process. While many believe that the weather-beaten 'Marlboro Man' look justifies giving up smoking, sun exposure is different because, as we shall see later, there are trade-off benefits with other bodily functions. However, this particular sun-and-smoking effect has nothing to do with the aging process.

The fundamental defect of skin aging is loss of collagen, the skin's main constituent, which is why aging skin thins. The loss is 1 per cent a year throughout adult life and is equal in men and women. The reason female skin appears to age faster than male is that women have less skin collagen to start with. The loss of collagen with age is genetic; it has absolutely nothing to do with UV irradiation and occurs equally in skin that has spent its life covered or exposed. And, contrary to the advertising blurb for anti-aging creams that simply irritate the skin producing inflammation that swells it and conceals the wrinkles, nothing is known that reverses this loss of collagen. Aging of the skin is *not* due to UV, and it *cannot* be overcome by the products of the cosmetic industry.

Skin cancer, however, is the big scare. The case that is made is that skin cancer is the commonest of all cancers and its increasing incidence is casually associated with solar irradiation. These facts are correct, but they have been mischievously interpreted. Indeed, the very word cancer is being deliberately used to create fear and coerce a public acceptance of these measures. Yet the key fact is that about 95 per cent of skin cancers are basal or squamous cell epitheliomas (the more minor basal cell variety making up about 85 per cent of the total) and, although they are called 'cancers', they are functionally benign: they do not spread from the skin and kill. Most are just a centimetre in size. A local excision is 95–99 per cent successful. Residual microscopic pieces of tumour disappear by themselves and the few recurrences are easily removed. The exceptions are rare and often the consequence of some other diseases. So, while 'skin cancer' is certainly the commonest cancer, the more honest statistic is that it is the least dangerous cancer: it lies at the very bottom of the mortality table.

So the problem of skin cancer shrivels as soon as you start to examine the problem because the vast majority of these lesions are benign. The problem is technical: these benign epitheliomas are classified as cancers from a particular appearance under the microscope, not from their behaviour. The public, for whom the word cancer creates fear, does not understand this. While it may be technically correct to say that skin cancer is related to sun exposure, this is meaningless because these sun-provoked lesions are not really cancers: they are small, local, slow growing and above all benign. These trivial benign lesions cannot possibly justify the aggressive hue and cry about avoidance of UV exposure. The misunderstanding has been inappropriately talked up by the Australian experience: the high incidence of skin cancer in Australia is the product of a high UV exposure in a population whose ancestors included many with pale, freckled skin and red hair. It should not be extrapolated to different populations living in sun-deprived climates.

But if skin cancer is the bait, melanoma is the hook. Melanoma is the least common of the three skin cancers. There is an alleged increase in its incidence and this is blamed on UV. People have been terrified into inspecting their skin regularly, even though it is of doubtful value. Most of us have simple moles and even more have seborrhoeic warts, which enlarge, get darker, itch and bleed in the same way as melanomas. Dermatological clinics are overfilled with patients worried about these totally innocent spots. Malignant melanomas are not found often enough to justify the hoo-ha about early screening, and there is no good evidence that screening saves lives.

Before pushing the clinical panic button, we should have had definite answers to two questions: is the increase in melanoma real, and what is its relationship to UV? Sadly, the answer to both questions is far too uncertain to justify what is being advised.

Certainly, there has been a big increase in reports of melanoma. The problem is that what is now being called melanoma may be nothing of the sort: it seems to be due to a reclassification of what constitutes malignancy. The diagnosis of malignancy in a melanoma is subjective; it's in the eye of the histopathologist looking down a microscope. In the past, it was commonplace for histopathologists to report borderline, minimal or dubiously suspicious histological appearances of moles. Experience of the outcome of these cases taught us that it was not alarming: we did nothing and nothing untoward happened to the patients. Later, as compensation claims began to dictate a more defensive practice, the same lesions started to be labelled suspicious, without the qualification of dubious. The process moved on, and it didn't take long before brown spots previously labelled benign acquired a new label indicating the possibility of early malignant change. In time, this moved on again to probability and finally to certainty. The moles have not changed, but the diagnosis has.

Having seen the process evolve, I have no doubt that re-labelling of benign lesions as malignant is a major, if not the main, cause of the increased incidence of reported malignant melanoma. I had confirmation of this from well-known clinicians who had observed the same development in other countries. But an idea is nothing without testing, and to put it to the test I proposed to send copies of the histology slides of moles that were labelled benign years ago from patients found by follow-up not to have had a malignant melanoma to a panel of histopathologists for their diagnosis by today's criteria. No laboratory would agree to take part in the study: although they agreed with its design, they appeared fearful of its outcome.

Support for this thesis comes from a variety of sources. The most important is that, while the incidence of melanoma has increased, it has not been accompanied by a corresponding change in mortality. In the UK, the annual number of melanomas in women increased by 250 per cent between 1980 and 2002, but the mortality from melanomas in women increased by just under 30 per cent and is decreasing. The reason for the apparent improvement is not that we have more effective therapy but that the number of cancers has been swollen by the new-wave melanomas. These have a cure rate of 100 per cent because they were never malignant in the first place: they are paper malignancies, benign moles reclassified. There are other explanations for the diagnostic confusion: for example, it is possible that UV, which is known to increase the number of moles, also induces changes that lead to them being classified as atypical, the jargon name for the features on which the histological diagnosis of malignancy may be based.

It has been found that death from melanoma is lower in the higher social classes. Does this mean that the genetic defect that causes the cancer is class related? This is obvious nonsense; the more likely reason is that the middle classes always turn up first and flock to the clinics with their benign moles which they have been frightened into having removed, and some of these are labelled malignant when in practice they are really benign. Until we have better diagnostic criteria, it is impossible to determine if the reported increase of malignant melanoma is genuine. The case for an increase in the prevalence of truly malignant melanoma remains unproven.

Even more doubtful is the role of UV as a causal agent. The evidence is fragile and certainly does not justify the present anti-solar terror campaign. What we might expect if UV really caused melanomas is illustrated by the skin epitheliomas. These cancers are caused by UV. They can be easily induced by UV in laboratory animals and in the case of epitheliomas there is an excellent correlation between their prevalence in patients, the latitude at which they live and between the site at which they occur and areas of the body exposed to UV. None of this is true of melanomas. Melanomas are difficult to produce experimentally, the correlation with the latitude at which the patients live is marginal, and their site of occurrence does not correspond to the intensity of its UV exposure. They are commonest on the trunks of men, the legs of women and the soles of the feet of Africans, a phenomenon not to be explained by exposure to the sun's rays. Their reported increase has been much less than the UV-related skin cancers and, unlike epitheliomas, there is no evidence that sunscreens prevent them from occurring.

The problem with melanoma, as with many other branches of contemporary clinical research, is that it is based on circumstantial evidence obtained from epidemiological studies rather than an understanding of the pathology. Melanoma is an illustration of the muddle introduced by uncritical acceptance of epidemiology, a preoccupation with which has distracted us from essential biology. For example, we still need to establish the melanoma's cell of origin. Is it a cancer of the pigment cell, the normal melanocyte, or does it start in the 'naevus' cell of a simple 'mole', which is something quite different? Establishing this is vital to our understanding because we know the distribution of moles over the skin surface but not naevus cells, let alone what makes them go malignant. It is well established that UV damage to DNA can produce cancer; but the only sensible conclusion from all the studies to date has to be that, while this effect plays a major role in producing epitheliomas, at worst it can only be marginal for melanomas. While UV is the main cause of epitheliomatous skin cancers, which are functionally benign, there is no hard evidence that UV is the principal cause of malignant melanomas.

What then should we do about UV exposure and sunscreens? The short answer is that, in moderate climates like the UK, apart from avoiding sunburn, it doesn't matter because the risk of exposure is trivial. Of course, children have to learn how much sun they can take without burning and their parents need to ensure they get a gradual UV exposure in order to achieve a protective tan – this is more important in children with ginger hair and freckles, most of whom will need to take care not to burn throughout adult life. In the UK, there is no point in trying to minimise sun exposure to avoid skin cancer because our sun is usually too weak to be a danger. Although sunscreens will reduce epithelioma formation, they have not been shown to prevent melanomas. The use of a sunblock in countries such as the UK could be harmful, because they impair vitamin D synthesis in the skin, increasing the risk of osteoporosis.

We still have a lot to learn about what may be the silent benefits of sun exposure. We do not know the significance and purpose of the profound changes in immune mechanisms, the extraordinary improvement in mood and the alleged decreased risk of bowel and prostatic cancer experienced after sun exposure. We may do more harm avoiding these advantages than anything we might gain from the uncertain benefits of sun avoidance. But not all of the sun's benefits are uncertain, particularly the protective effect of a suntan. Since there is some epidemiological evidence to suggest that sunburn in children may be more harmful later in life, parents have been told that sun exposure must be avoided in childhood. However, if you take a close look at people who were sunburned as children, you will see areas of white skin that doesn't tan because the pigment cells have been lost. Such skin will always be oversensitive to sun. It is evident that the original sunburn, and subsequent damage, would have been less had there already been a protective tan. Excessive avoidance and UV screening is a danger because it does not allow a tan, nature's own sunblock, to develop and as a result exposure is likely to cause sunburn. The dogma, now fossilised in print, is that any tan is a sign of skin damage; this is intuitively improbable. Pigmented melanocytes in the skin are part of a system that evolved to protect long before the advent of dermatologists and sunscreens. Even if there was hard evidence that melanoma was UV induced, it would be all the more important to keep a protective tan.

It must now be evident that the effect of the sun on the skin is in desperate need of illumination, and that the prophylactic message, particularly for melanoma, is unreliable. Regardless of how and why this sorry situation arose, the hope is that awareness of the fragility of the epidemiological case against UVR will lead to more solid scientific study, after which prophylaxis can be based on reality rather than pseudo-scientific myth.

Chapter Twenty-one

SCREENING FOR BREAST CANCER

BY MICHAEL BAUM

The Myth: **Breast-cancer screening saves tens of thousands of lives.**
The Fact: **Breast-cancer screening is unlikely to catch fatal cancers.**

Every year we have breast cancer awareness month, or what I choose to call Black October. Each October in the UK, women are advised to practise breast self-examination (a thoroughly discredited practice)* and are reminded that their risk of developing the disease is 1 in 11. This number is true only if a woman outlives all other competing risks to her health and reaches the age of 85; in fact, 25 out of every 26 women die of other causes before this age. It is essential therefore that both doctors and the public understand the risk of developing breast cancer in the various age groups, and understand the expectation of life after the diagnosis of breast cancer both with and without screening.

---

* Three large national trials (UK, Russia and China) have compared breast-cancer death rates amongst women taught breast self-examination (BSE) and those left to their own devices. Amongst the tens of thousands of women in these studies there was no difference in breast-cancer mortality but those taught BSE suffered twice the number of unnecessary biopsies.

One must consider the various forms of bias inherent in any analysis of the value of mammographic screening that support my somewhat counter-intuitive view that screening is not all that it's cracked up to be.

BIASES IN SCREENING

Lead-time Bias

Say you get on a train going to Edinburgh. Before it reaches its destination it crashes. The duration of your fatal journey depends on your departure point. If you board the train at Milton Keynes, half an hour's train journey from London, your expectation of survival before the fatal crash would be two and a half hours, whereas if you left from Kings Cross it would have been three hours. No matter where you started, you still die at the same time. In a similar way, merely shifting the period of observation of breast cancer will alter the survival time from the point of diagnosis, without necessarily extending the duration of your life.

Length bias

Say you trawl the sea for fish with a slow boat. You will catch the slow fish but miss those that can swim faster than your trawler. By the same token, if you trawl the female population for breast cancer at intervals you will catch the slow-growing cancers, the ones that are likely to have been cured anyway if allowed to grow to a clinically detectable stage, while missing the rapidly growing cancers that occur in the intervals between screening – and these are probably the ones that will kill you.

Class Bias

Not all women invited for screening are 'compliant' and accept the invitation. The better off, who are health conscious, tend to accept, while the poorer ones often ignore the request or never get it in the first place because they are of no fixed abode. This affects the results of surveys of the effectiveness of screening, since we know that the outcome of treatment, stage for stage, is better among the affluent.

THE TRIALS OF SCREENING AND RELATIVE RISK REDUCTIONS

To get round these problems and assess the value of screening, it is necessary to carry out randomised trials in whole populations with the outcome measure being breast-cancer mortality.

There have been eight randomised or quasi-randomised trials of population mammographic screening for breast cancer. In addition, there have been a number of attempts to conduct a meta-analysis of all these studies to increase the numbers. Finally, there was the Cochrane Review, which attempted to weight the studies for quality to overcome the defects of meta-analysis before providing a summary statistic. This study was published by Olsen and Gotzche in the *Lancet* in 2001. It provoked the editor of the *Lancet*, Richard Horton, to state: 'At present there is no reliable evidence from large randomised trials to support mammography programmes.'

Whatever the merits or flaws in the Cochrane Review, a number of unassailable facts emerged. The Canadian study was the only one that was properly randomised and it did not show any positive beneficial effect from screening. The HIP study from New York, which produced the most favourable result, excluded three times as many patients in the screened group compared with the control group on the grounds that they were 'unsatisfactory due to a history of cancer'. The Edinburgh trial, which was randomised according to postal district, ended up with huge imbalances in socio-economic factors favouring those in the higher-income groups in the screened population. In these trials, the best effect of screening appeared to have been in those centres using the worst equipment and the longest screening intervals. This suggests that there are problems underlying the interpretation of these results.

All these trials failed to show a truly proven effect of screening that stands up to scientific scrutiny.

Let us consider the more optimistic estimates produced by two overview analyses, a Swedish study and the US preventive services task force 2002. Neither could show a significant advantage for women under the age of 50 (in fact, the latest result from the

Canadian trial for the under-50 group actually showed a worse result for the first 10 years), whereas their estimates for the over-50 age group demonstrated a relative risk reduction between 16 per cent and 25 per cent for death from cancer of the breast. Let us now examine just what that means in absolute terms in an individual woman over the 10-year period of the study.

The risk of a woman aged 50–60 developing breast cancer is 2 in 1,000 per year, or 2 per cent over a decade (20 out of 1,000). The anticipated 10-year survival for clinically detected breast cancer in the absence of screening today is about 75 per cent. Therefore, we can expect five deaths per thousand women from breast cancer over a 10-year period (75 per cent of 20 per cent). The relative risk reduction for screening only applies to these five women. A realistic estimate would be that screening might save one life in a thousand, while 999 women have to share the side-effects and the cost.

THE DOWN SIDE OF SCREENING

In all imperfect screening tools, there is a balance between the sensitivity of the test and its specificity. Sensitivity is a measure of the ability to detect the cancers, whereas specificity is a measure of the accuracy of the screening tool. These two measures tend to pull in opposite directions. One hundred per cent sensitivity implies not missing a single cancer. To achieve this, the specificity will inevitably fall, and many women with benign changes on mammography will have their breast biopsied. There always has to be a delicate balance between these opposing needs – the ideal of detecting all the cancers while protecting women without cancer from false alarms and unnecessary invasive procedures. Even in the very best centres, for every woman who has a cancer detected, another woman will have a false alarm. Because of the fear of litigation, there is a tendency to be cautious, with the result that any unclear case is labelled as a possible cancer.

The cumulative risk of a false alarm over the past decade of screening has risen to around 40 per cent. This results in unnecessary patient anxiety, and in surgery that has its own morbidity and tends to throw up pathology of uncertain, borderline significance. The public can be forgiven for thinking that a pathologist can make a clear distinction between cancer and non-cancer, but sadly that is not the case. There is a whole spectrum of conditions labelled as carcinoma, many of uncertain significance and unknown natural history. A conservative estimate would suggest that less than half of these would threaten a woman's life if left undetected, and yet they account for 20 per cent of the 'cancers' detected at screening.

Next there is the issue of 'lead time'. At one end of the spectrum, we can consider the woman with her cancer detected at screening who is doomed to die, while at the other end is the women with a cancer that would have been cured even if left for one to two years, when the lump would have made a clinical diagnosis inevitable. Any study incorporating both women would find that the latter patient's life expectancy was longer and attribute this to screening.

Finally, women invited for screening should be aware that the detection of a possible cancer of the breast, with all the uncertainties described above, might have an effect on the premiums for their health or life insurance.

ETHICAL ISSUES

Modern medicine is a minefield of ethical dilemmas. When analysing these problems, the scholarly medical ethicist tends to fall back on the teachings of Immanuel Kant and his concepts of the categorical imperatives of human relationships in a democratic society:

> Finally, there is an imperative which commands a certain conduct immediately, without having as its condition any other purpose to be attained by it. This imperative is categorical. This imperative may be called that of morality.
> *Grundlegung zur Metaphysik der Sitten,* section II

These imperatives, known as the four principles, can be listed as follows:

Beneficence (the obligation to provide benefits and balance benefits against risks)

Non-maleficence (the obligation to avoid the causation of harm)

Respect for autonomy (the obligation to respect the decision-making capacities of autonomous persons)

Justice (the obligation of fairness in the distribution of benefits and risks)

I would like to add a fifth:

Distributive justice (the obligation to ensure that scarce resources are distributed fairly among the health services for the greatest health improvement for the greatest number)

This 'utilitarian' principle is an extension of the teachings of Jeremy Bentham (1748–1832), the founder of University College London, who argued for the greatest good for the greatest number: 'Everybody to count for one, nobody for more than one.' Unfortunately, it is never easy to achieve a moral equilibrium. The greatest ethical dilemmas in medicine follow on from a clash of these ethical imperatives.

It is my contention that the subject of screening for breast cancer has been allowed to drift into accepted public health practice without an appropriate ethical debate. In discussing the ethical issues of screening for cancer, we must accept a tension that exists between utilitarian principles of public health and the principle of the autonomy of the individual. Utilitarianism involves the 'greatest good of the greatest number', whereas autonomy assumes that the individual has an informed choice when health interventions for 'their own good' are considered. Nowhere is this more true than in the area of mammographic screening for breast cancer. We screen for breast cancer to reduce the mortality at an acceptable cost, in terms of medical morbidity. At the same time, we should also consider whether the costs of such programmes might be spent in better ways – could the resources be better used to improve healthcare in the community? Even if we accept uncritically the results of the randomised controlled trials, the reduction in death from breast cancer is so small (widely accepted as 1:10,000 woman years in screening over the age of 50 and about 1:15,000 woman years in screening for the younger age groups) that the individual woman should have the right to make a personal trade-off against the undoubted risks of breast biopsy and the anxieties caused by a false alarm in cases where the tumour, if left to nature, would never announce itself in a natural lifetime.

The uncritical promotion of the benefits of breast screening by high-profile government campaigns is unethical by modern standards and reflects a paternalistic attitude that would be unacceptable in the treatment of any established disease.

Finally, in the name of distributive justice I believe that, in the UK at least, we should have an open debate about the £50 million a year that is spent on the National Health Service breast-screening programme. This money might be better used by a more focused approach to the disease or on post-operative therapies. I have a sneaking suspicion that there is a political agenda here, not only for the UK but also for the rest of Europe. Screening demonstrates that the government is working for women and 'doing something about breast cancer', whereas other uses of the same money will not win votes.

WHERE DO WE GO FROM HERE?

I believe that, now that we know the full costs and benefits of screening, to carry on complacently is not an option. However, I see a decision to end screening as politically impossible, so the best I could hope for here might be a shift in the screening window to the 55–69 age group, where sensitivity and specificity might be improved.

If nothing else, I believe there is an ethical imperative to offer women full, informed consent before they have their breasts screened. The risk and benefits should be spelled out in terms that don't patronise or deceive them. If, after that, the women vote with their feet, so be it.

Chapter Twenty-two

STRESS AND ILLNESS –
A MODERN DISEASE?

BY PAUL R GROB

'Let no one persuade you to cure the headache until he has
first given you his soul to be cured. For this is the great error of
our day in the treatment of the human body, that physicians
separate the soul from the body.'

HIPPOCRATES, 2002 BC

The Myth: **The stress of the society in which we live has developed a whole new range
of illnesses.**
The Fact: **A substantial proportion of these 'illnesses' in fact have other causes.**

We live in an age of uncertainty. People are concerned about the
effect of GM crops. Is the MMR vaccine safe? Will we be
attacked by terrorists? Is it safe to fly? Thus, all these facts amplify
the natural concerns about how we should conduct our lives. This
background of uncertainty heightens our natural concern and spills
over into our belief that stress is a major component of many of the
illnesses we experience today.

Stress is said to be due to the pace of modern living and is generally thought of as being harmful. However, stress has been vital for our survival since the dawn of time. The body's reaction to stress, the adrenaline response, is 'hard-wired' into our physiology and accounts for our increased performance when our survival is threatened.

To a hunter-gatherer animal such as man, stress is a way of life, whereas, to a white landrace pig, stress literally turns its flesh to jelly. To an athlete preparing for a 100-metre race, stress is helpful and enhances his performance – recognition of this effect has led to the banning of drugs that simulate the stress response. To one actor preparing for his first night, stress may cause stage fright, whereas in another it may elevate his performance to a new level. To a businessman awaiting bankruptcy, it causes depression and sleeplessness, whereas, to an Arctic explorer on a mountain ledge, stress is part of his existence and he will sleep soundly. To a worker who finds his job beyond his capability, stress causes anxiety, restlessness and ill health. In all of these circumstances the stress response is the same; it is the way the body interprets it that determines whether or not it does us any harm.

To understand stress, it is necessary to step back and examine the evolution of our behavioural patterns. Early life forms were merely capable of reacting passively to changes in the world around them. They moved away from inhospitable environments, closed their carapace or rolled into tight balls when in danger. A primitive brain controlled these functions. Once more advanced forms of life that were capable of searching for food, escaping from danger and fighting to protect their young evolved, a more sophisticated control system was required. This was reflected in the development of a new part of the brain that could co-ordinate information and evoke appropriate responses. To prepare for any subsequent exertion it needed a system to increase the energy level in the cells of the body so as to make it ready for action. This function was carried out by the sympathetic nervous system, the so-called 'fight-or-flight' system. An essential component of this system was that of the adrenal glands (really two glands stuck together on top of the kidneys) which pumped out adrenalin and steroids into the blood stream. It is the outpouring of these hormones that we measure as the stress response.

We are continually battling with events that destabilise the way we live. The strain imposed upon life by destabilising circumstances (stressors) causes a complex spectrum of physiological and behavioural responses that try to restore stability. Failure of the living organism to adapt to stress results in death; life's adaptation to a constantly changing environment has been essential for evolution.

Stress can be motivating, bringing forth excellence in an individual, but stress that is unrelenting can be detrimental to health. Research has shown that there are health benefits involved in performing exciting projects and hustling to meet occasional deadlines. The stress hormones released in times of pressure can increase creativity in one person, while in another the same hormones will cause anxiety and depression.

There is no simple way of predicting what will cause harmful levels of stress as people respond to different stressors in different, unpredictable ways. Levi in 1992 pointed out that the feeling of 'being in control' and 'on top of the job at hand' determined whether people felt that a particular stress was the spice of life or a threat. When this crucial sense of control is lacking, stress will have an adverse effect on the individual.

There is a growing body of evidence that suggests that prolonged periods of stress may cause a wide spectrum of diverse illnesses. Those relationships are at their most convincing when the stressors relate particularly to adverse life events and major changes in, or intensity of, work and working relationships. Most people can relate to the experience of getting sick at an inopportune time when they are under stress and there is a lot to do. As Freud said, no accidents are accidental: it is interesting to note how often an accident or illness occurs when the body is in need of rest and recuperation. If stress plays a role in the acquisition of minor ailments, what then is its effect on the cause of major diseases?

A great deal of research has been done to determine the role of stress on the development of diseases. Cardiovascular disorders, gastrointestinal disease and certain neurological disorders are among those physical illnesses in which links to stress feature prominently. These relationships can be identified in epidemiological surveys and controlled studies, the relative risk of their occurrence is highly variable and the findings cannot readily be extrapolated to the individual person. Only rarely can a specific factor be teased out to establish a causal relationship for chronic stressors in an individual case.

So how much does stress contribute to illness in our modern-day society? It is clearly an area of great concern as there are over 15 million websites on the Internet related to stress and life and this must represent a deep-seated 'angst' felt in our modern society. We all recognise that stress over a prolonged period generates an unpleasant state of anxiety which is characterised by fearfulness, sleeplessness, depression and unwanted and distressing physical symptoms. Anxiety disorders such as panic attacks, phobic states and obsessive-compulsive disorders seem to be exacerbated or initiated by chronic stress.

Post-traumatic stress disorder (PTSD) has been recognised for many years. It describes emotional and physical disorders that follow a traumatic experience that is outside the normal field of human expectation. Although it is recognised as an understandable response to specific conditions, its full ramifications and long-term effects are difficult to predict, particularly when litigation, compensation and benefit are at issue. In recent times there has been an enormous increase in the number of patients purporting to be suffering from this condition, although there is little doubt that the number of those claiming to suffer from PTSD and the severity of their symptoms are increased when there is prospect of significant compensation. People who have not actually witnessed a trauma first-hand become involved and experience the symptoms of the illness. This has led to considerable cynicism as to the true incidence of the syndrome. In a study of veterans of the Vietnam War, Dr Pankratz of the University of Oregon found that less than 20 per cent of those receiving compensation for PTSD had actually witnessed any fighting. It is difficult to understand why those who have not witnessed the horrors of war first-hand should be more commonly affected than those who have. Similarly, those who have survived life in a concentration camp may suffer nightmares, anxiety states and depression, but they seldom exhibit the physical symptoms of PTSD.

In order to limit exposure to litigation from patients suffering from PTSD, it is now usual to offer counselling when a person is subjected to an unpleasant experience. This has spawned an industry of counselling and, while it may be comforting to some, there is little evidence of its general efficacy. Post-traumatic stress may provoke the onset of clinical depression. Brown in 1989 clearly demonstrated that a substantial proportion of patients with a recent onset of a depressive disorder had experienced an adverse life event, particularly one involving loss or separation, during the six months preceding the onset of the depressive symptoms. This is particularly true in women.

Chronic fatigue syndrome (CFS) is now the preferred term for a variety of different conditions including post-viral fatigue and myalgic encephalomyelitis (ME). The opinion of the medical profession is fairly evenly split over the cause of this syndrome. Many believe it to be a stress-related depression, while others hold the view that it is a physical illness whose cause or causes are unknown. The term 'chronic fatigue' makes no assumptions about the cause of the syndrome. It is unusual for patients with this debilitating condition to have any demonstrable blood or neurological changes. Many people with this syndrome exhibit a particular type of personality and follow highly demanding, stressful lifestyles, which suggests that occupational stress may have a part in causing this condition.

The effect of stress, personality and heart disease has long been recognised. Cardiac symptoms, in those in whom there appeared to be no specific heart disease, were catalogued and explored during the Crimean War, and were also reported in soldiers during the American

Civil War. More recent studies have shown that there is a considerably increased frequency of heart attacks in the hour or so after heavy physical exertion. There is some evidence of an increased risk of a myocardial infarction following an emotional upset or acute psychological stress. The association between lifestyles and raised blood pressure has been clearly recognised. This is to be expected as adrenalin, the principal hormone of the stress response, raises the blood pressure. A change of lifestyle or working environment may help in reducing the blood pressure and relieving symptoms.

An increasing frequency of epileptic seizures during periods of physical or psychological stress has been reported on numerous occasions by those who suffer from the condition. However, there may be other important contributory factors, such as lack of sleep, alcohol consumption, omitting drug therapy and, perhaps most importantly, involuntary hyperventilation.

The link between psychological factors and the occurrence of various forms of cancer has been an intriguing source of speculation. However, anecdotal stories of cancer following a stressful event have not been supported by careful investigation. More reasonable attention has been focused on the possibility of an association between breast cancer and stress. The association, if it is present, is thought to involve the individual's predisposition and a range of potential stressors, balanced by the response of the individual, the effect on the immune system and various different support systems.

We all have experienced the gastrointestinal effects of acute stress. The expression 'sick with fear' has meaning as virtually everybody has experienced this symptom from time to time. The dry mouth and stomach cramps of the actor on the first night of a play are well documented. Psychological factors have traditionally been associated with the causation and relapse of irritable bowel syndrome and sufferers from this condition often recognise the precipitating effect of lifestyle stresses. There is a traditionally held view that ulcerative colitis, a particularly debilitating and distressing condition, has a strong psychosomatic element. However, others have held the view that it is the constant watery diarrhoea that produces the personality change in the victim. The disease is found in the type of person who readily responds to emotional disturbance. The diarrhoea often becomes worse after a stressful, emotional event.

Asthma attacks are often precipitated by a stressful event. This is not always obvious. A patient of mine kept a daily record of the severity of his asthma and then linked it to life events. It became clear after some time that his asthma got much worse at the end of the month when meetings to discuss his sales targets took place. Appreciation of this linkage was a major factor in producing an improvement of his condition.

How can we minimise our response to the inevitable stress of modern living? Clausewitz, a Prussian military writer, always insisted that the first step in any campaign was securing your base camp. In everyday, life this means a secure home environment with its associated love and support. Research has shown that the effect of stress can be reduced by developing this resilience. We seem to be able to cope, by and large, with major threats to our existence such as loss, bereavement and separation, but it is the minor, unrelenting trials of life that eventually wear us down.

Two guidelines are useful in dealing with stress. First, listen to the messages your body is giving you. Physical and mental fatigue are often signs of chronic stress and, if your body wants to go to sleep or rest, pay attention to this message. Second, be kind to yourself. We all develop a picture of how we should behave in order to succeed in life. This is our 'cage of duty' – go to work, get the children off to school, do the shopping, look after the family and so on. The key that unlocks our 'cage of duty' is within the cage itself and we can use it to escape. The realisation that we have not necessarily to accept the straitjacket of behaviour imposed on us by our 'duty' to society may be a life-changing event.

Chapter Twenty-three

THE SMOKESCREEN OF PASSIVE SMOKING

BY JAMES LEFANU

The Myth: Passive smoking causes lung cancer.

The Fact: The claim that passive smoking causes lung cancer is statistically improbable and biologically implausible.

The British government's recent commitment to enforce a smoking ban in offices, restaurants and most public houses is without doubt a decisive victory in the long protracted battle against the evils of tobacco. Until very recently the proposal to prohibit smoking would have been met with the rejoinder 'You must be joking!' But now the deed is done, and in retrospect the ban, like the drink-driving law and the compulsory wearing of seatbelts, now seems mere commonsense. Indeed, even those who would be expected to oppose it as a 'step too far' in curtailing individual freedom seem reconciled – as the erstwhile Shadow Arts Minister Boris Johnson recently observed in an article in the *Daily Telegraph*:

'And I tell you this, gentlemen,' I said and one hundred golfers in black tie boggled drunkenly and hung upon my words ... 'you know what this Labour government wants to ban?' I yipped.

'What?' they chorused, red faced with anticipatory wrath. 'They want to stop you – smoking!' I said. 'No more smoking in the workplace, or pubs, or restaurants; no more pint 'n' Castella at the nineteenth hole, and so far as the putting green is a public place, you will probably be forbidden even from having a crafty fag as you steady your nerves!'

'Outrageous' they said, and for a while the surf of indignation thundered around me, until a man just to my right piped up in level tones: 'Well, you know, I am all in favour of a ban, actually.'

'What?' I said, amazed, but before I could get to the bottom of his dissent, two or three others around the room were putting their hands up and demanding a ban on any kind of smoking in public ... the honest truth, they said, was that they used to be smokers themselves, and it was a filthy habit, and they thought the new law would help them to resist any temptation to take it up again.

The argument that 'won it' for the ban on smoking in bars and restaurants was the claim that passive smoking (also known as 'Environmental Tobacco Smoke' (ETS)) is not merely offensive to others but potentially as injurious to the health of innocent bystanders as active smoking is for smokers themselves. The relevant scientific evidence, in the aftermath of the government's ban, may seem merely of historic interest, but nonetheless merits critical scrutiny as an instructive example of how medical researchers manipulate evidence for what they believe to be a legitimate political goal. Or, as a public-health specialist confided to the distinguished epidemiologist the late Professor Alvin Feinstein of Yale University, 'It is rotten science, but in a worthy cause. It will help us get rid of cigarettes to become a smoke-free society. That is all that really matters.' How did they do it?

Back in 1988 the Environmental Protection Agency (EPA) resolved to lobby the US government to ban smoking in public as a preliminary move in its long-term goal of outlawing it altogether. It was likely, however, to be difficult to prove the injurious effects of passive smoking if for no other reason than that non-smokers are only exposed, in relative terms, to minuscule amounts of tobacco smoke – estimated at around the equivalent of actively smoking six cigarettes per year. Nonetheless, a group of researchers came up with the ingenious proposal comparing the rates of lung cancer and heart disease in the non-smoking wives of smoking husbands with those where neither partner smoked, which might show passive smoking to be a factor in at least some cases. Their findings, as might be expected, were equivocal: some studies did show a small positive effect, while others, perversely, showed that women married to a smoking husband might even be protected against lung cancer. Or even that passive smoking was more dangerous than active smoking – with one study showing that the non-smoking wives of heavy smokers had a higher rate of lung cancer than active smokers.

So, there was not much support here for the supposedly carcinogenic effects of passive smoking – and the evidence for its dangers seemed tenuous for another reason: the cases of lung cancer that were identified in these studies were not those normally associated with active smoking. To explain. There are two broad categories of lung cancer, the commonest (Group 1) being squamous and oat cell cancers that arise from the cells lining the airways (that are maximally exposed to the potential carcinogens in tobacco smoke). The second type (Group 2) is known as adenocarcinomas which arise from glandular tissue in the air sacs in the periphery of the lung.

Back in the early 1950s, when the late Sir Austin Bradford Hill first produced the powerful evidence implicating active smoking in lung cancer, he made the important observation that these tobacco-induced cancers were exclusively of the Group 1-type – squamous and oat cell cancers where (as shown in *Figure 5*) there is a powerful dose–response relationship, where with the more smoked, the greater the risks. By contrast he could find no association between smoking and Group 2-type adenocarcinomas (as shown by the flat line at the bottom of the graph) reflecting the absence of any biological gradient from which it would be reasonable to infer that whatever might be their cause it has nothing to do with smoking.

So, if passive smoking was indeed the cause of some cases of lung cancer in the studies sponsored by the EPA, it was necessary to presuppose the following: that carcinogenic smoke as inhaled by active smokers over many years causes squamous and oat cell cancers to the airways, but the same smoke when inhaled by passive smokers at almost infinitely lower doses causes an entirely different type of cancer (adenocarcinomas) in a different part of the lung that is not associated with active smoking. This is, to put it mildly, highly improbable.

Clearly, the protagonists of the evils of passive smoking must have deployed some ingenious statistical alchemy to transform this sow's ear of contradictory studies and biological implausibility into the silk purse of the 'compelling evidence' that would eventually cause the British government to ban smoking in public places.

It is helpful in answering this conundrum to remind ourselves of the original evidence implicating active smoking in lung cancer. Sir Austin Bradford Hill devised two separate but complementary methods by which to establish whether an environmental phenomenon (such as tobacco) might cause some disease (say lung cancer).

The first of these was the Cohort Study which requires assessing the social habits of a defined group of people, and following them up over a long period to see whether those habits correlate with their subsequent cause of death. The most famous of these Cohort Studies was Sir Austin's own 'doctor's study' in which every doctor in Britain was invited to report their smoking habits and which, over the next forty years, revealed that the smokers amongst them had an unequivocal twenty-fivefold increased risk of lung cancer.

FIGURE 5

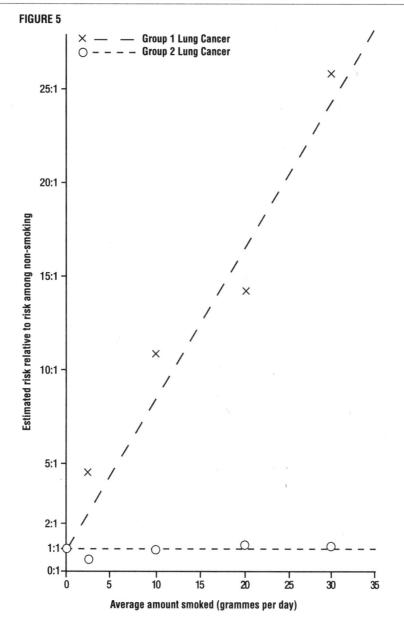

X — — Group 1 Lung Cancer
O – – – – Group 2 Lung Cancer

Biologically implausible: Smoking causes Group 1 lung cancers, shown by diagonal dose–response relationship, where the more smoked, the greater the risk. The absence of the same biological gradient, with Group 2 carcinomas (flat line) is strong evidence against their being caused by passive smoking.

His second epidemiological method was the Case-Control Study where the social habits of a group of patients with the disease of interest is compared with a control group and any obvious differences can then be inferred as a putative cause of that disease.

FIGURE 6

Study	Year, country	Women Lung cancer cases	Controls	Relative risk (95% confidence interval)	Men Lung cancer cases	Controls	Relative risk (95% confidence interval)
Case-control sudies							
Chan et al	1982, Hong Kong	84	139	0.75 (0.43 to 1.30)			
Correa et al	1983, USA	22	133	2.07 (0.81 to 5.25)	8	180	1.97 (0.38 to 0.32)
Trichopolous et al	1983, Greece	62	190	2.13 (1.19 to 3.83)			
Buffler et al	1984, USA	41	196	0.80 (0.34 to 1.90)	11	90	0.51 (0.14 to 1.79)
Kabat et al	1984, USA	24	25	0.79 (0.25 to 2.45)	12	12	1.00 (0.10 to 5.07)
Lam	1985, Hong Kong	60	144	2.01 (1.09 to 3.72)			
Garfinkel et al	1985, USA	134	402	1.23 (0.81 to 1.87)			
Wu et al	1985, USA	29	62	1.20 (0.50 to 3.30)			
Akiba et al	1986, Japan	94	270	1.52 (0.87 to 2.63)	19	110	2.10 (0.51 to 8.61)
Lee et al	1986, UK	32	66	1.03 (0.41 to 2.55)	15	30	1.31 (0.38 to 4.52)
Koo et al	1987, Hong Kong	86	136	1.55 (0.90 to 2.67)			
Pershagen et al	1987, Sweden	70	294	1.03 (0.61 to 1.74)			
Humble et al	1987, USA	20	162	2.34 (0.81 to 6.75)			
Lam et al	1987, Hong Kong	199	335	1.65 (1.16 to 2.35)			
Gao et al	1987, China	246	375	1.19 (0.82 to 1.73)			
Brownson et al	1987, USA	19	47	1.52 (0.39 to 5.96)			
Geng et al	1988, China	54	93	2.16 (1.08 to 4.29)			
Shimizu et al	1988, Japan	90	163	1.08 (0.64 to 1.82)			
Inoue et al	1988, Japan	22	47	2.55 (0.74 to 8.78)			
Kalandidi et al	1990, Greece	90	116	1.62 (0.90 to 2.91)			
Sobue	1990, Japan	144	731	1.06 (0.74 to 1.52)			
Wu-Williams et al	1990, China	417	602	0.79 (0.62 to 1.02)			
Liu et al	1991, China	54	202	0.74 (0.32 to 1.69)			
Jockel	1991, Germany	23	45	2.27 (0.75 to 6.82)	9	70	2.68 (0.58 to 12.36)
Brownson et al	1992, USA	431	1166	0.97 (0.78 to 1.21)			
Stockwell et al	1992, USA	210	301	1.60 (0.80 to 3.00)			
Du et al	1993, China	75	128	1.19 (0.66 to 2.13)			
Liu et al	1993, China	38	69	1.66 (0.73 to 3.78)			
Fontham et al	1994, USA	651	1253	1.26 (1.04 to 1.54)			
Kabat et al	1995, USA	67	173	1.10 (0.62 to 1.96)	39	98	1.63 (0.69 to 3.85)
Zaridze et al	1995, Russia	162	285	1.66 (1.12 to 2.45)			
Sun et al	1996, China	230	230	1.16 (0.80 to 1.69)			
Wang et al	1996, China	135	135	1.11 (0.67 to 1.84)			
Cohort studies							
Garfinkel	1981, USA	153	176586	1.18 (0.90 to 1.54)			
Hirayama	1984, Japan	200	91340	1.45 (1.02 to 2.08)	64	20225	2.25 (1.06 to 4.76)
Butler	1988, USA	8	9199	2.02 (0.48 to 8.56)			
Cardenas et al	1997, USA	150	192084	1.20 (0.80 to 1.60)	97	96445	1.00 (0.60 to 1.80)
All studies (37 studies of women, 9 studies of men)*							
	1981-97	4626	477924	1.24 (1.13 to 1.36) (P<0.001)	274	117260	1.34 (0.97 to 1.84) (P=0.07)

Statistically implausible: The summary of the 37 studies investigating passive smoking and lung cancer looks very impressive but fails to show the contradictory findings of the Case-Control Studies and the crucial negative findings of the American Cancer Society's massive Cohort Study.

Here again Sir Austin (as already shown in *Figure 5*) was able to identify a close dose–response relationship, where the more smoked, the greater the subsequent risk of lung cancer (though only of the Group 1-type).

Self-evidently, the fact that both forms of investigation came to the same conclusion is very significant as they show the evidence linking smoking and lung cancer to be internally highly coherent. This is, as it were, the 'gold standard' of epidemiological proof.

We turn now to examine the findings of these two different methods in investigating the putative link between passive smoking and lung cancer as summarised by Nicholas Wald, Professor of Epidemiology at St Bartholomew's Hospital, in the *BMJ* in 1997 (see *Figure 6*).

This massive synthesis of all the 'accumulated evidence' – 37 Case-Control and Cohort Studies revealed an impressive 26 per cent increased risk of lung cancer. Professor Wald's personal view that this was 'compelling' evidence was echoed by others such as Dr David Burns of the University of California who claimed in the *Journal of the National Cancer Institute* that 'the causal relationship between Environmental Tobacco Smoke and lung cancer is now firmly established'.

Now this was all very surprising because we have already noted the highly equivocal findings of many of those Case-Control Studies, while the fact that the lung cancers were of a different histological type to those associated with active smoking would suggest that a causative link was highly improbable. Clearly, it is necessary to take a closer look at that impressive-looking table.

First, we note how most of the Case-Control Studies come from countries such as Japan and China where the epidemiology of lung cancer is different from the West, with a particularly high incidence of those (non-smoking-related) adenocarcinomas. Then, we find, moving over to the heading 'Relative Risk' and scanning downwards the contradictory results already alluded to: some (where the risk is less than one) demonstrate a protective effect for passive smoking; most hovering around the no-effects level of one, while a minority show an increased risk of twofold or more.

We find a similar pattern when examining the four Cohort Studies, but if we look closely at the last and most recent – a massive project conducted by the American Cancer Society with nearly a quarter of a million men and women – we see the results range between the minuscule (1.20) to no effect (1.0) in men and women respectively.

This final Cohort Study is clearly by far the most significant of all in the table, but its very important findings disproving the carcinogenic effect of passive smoking have, as it were, been obliterated by combining it with all the Case-Control Studies, some of whose 'highly significant results' are sufficient to produce the 'overall' effect of the increased risk of 25%.

Nor is that all. When it comes to epidemiological studies it is a matter of 'the bigger the better' so one substantial Case-Control study carried a lot more weight than the many small contradictory studies, mostly from the Far East, sited in the table. The following year, the World Health Organisation concluded just such a megastudy – but its results were never published as they found 'no association between lung cancer risk and exposure to environmental tobacco smoke'.

So the question whether passive smoking really does cause lung cancer depends on what sort of evidence one finds the more convincing. The answer is yes if you believe the 'positive' results of Professor Wald's meta-analysis whose inclusion of many small studies from the Far East concealed the outcome of the American Cancer Society's Cohort Study. The answer is 'no' if you accept the 'negative' results of two massive studies of different design (the American Cancer Society's Cohort study and the WHO Case-Control Study) – though the findings of the former, as has been noted, were somewhat obscured, and the latter not included. To be sure, the former carried the day but common sense, logic and reasonable judgement would favour the latter. Professor Wald's meta-analysis became the much sought-after 'proof' that passive smoking was harmful to innocent bystanders – thus providing the scientific rationale for the subsequent proposal to ban smoking in offices, restaurants and most pubs. But the creative statistics involved were all in a good cause – so it doesn't really matter.

Chapter Twenty-four

CURRENT THOUGHTS ON THE SAFETY OF HRT

BY JOHN STUDD

The Myth: **HRT presents a huge number of health risks.**

The Fact: **There is no evidence to suggest there is any significant health risk from HRT; indeed, there are a number or well-documented health benefits.**

The history of clinical medicine is strewn with fashionable treatments supported by the experts, the unscrupulous or the downright eccentric, which have subsequently been discredited to become an odd footnote to medical history. The many biochemical placental function tests and surgical ventrosuspension for all cases of infertility are but a few examples in gynaecology. We must not forget that bleeding for anaemia was fashionable for centuries. Will this be the fate of hormone replacement therapy (HRT) for problems related to the menopause?

Over the last 20 years it has been believed that HRT has a hugely beneficial effect on post-menopausal women, without being complicated by many major side-effects. There was an anxiety that it could cause a very small increase in breast cancer but, as the survival rate was very much greater in women receiving HRT, it was easy to believe that it was not a major problem and that possibly the apparent increase was the result of overstimulation of breast cancer with oestrogens rather than a new malignancy. It was believed that oestrogens not only treated the hot flushes, insomnia, vaginal dryness and depression that occurred around the time of the menopause, but also that it prevented many heart attacks, strokes, colon cancer, Alzheimer's disease and osteoporotic fractures of the spine and the hip. There was also good evidence that women on HRT lived about 2.5 years longer, hopefully in a state of increased independence, with less dementia or Alzheimer's disease.

There was always little doubt that these optimistic observational studies were biased, because physicians would tend to give oestrogens to healthy, thin, non-diabetic, non-hypertensive, non-smoking, low-risk women. But the enthusiasm was such that in some countries, particularly the United States, oestrogens were given out to as many as 50 per cent of the aged female population in order to prevent strokes and dementia. It is for this reason that a huge randomised trial – the Women's Health Initiative (WHI) – was set up, to test the hypothesis that oestrogen therapy prevented these cardiovascular complications.

Almost 20,000 women were recruited from the age of 50–79, with the average age being 63 and 23 per cent being over the age of 70. In the UK, 96 per cent of our patients start HRT below the age of 60. The women in the WHI study were given conjugated equine oestrogens (Premarin). This is the major oestrogen used in the USA, but it is used much less frequently in Europe, where the natural human oestradiol by tablet, patch, gel, intra-nasal spray or implant is preferred. The patients in the WHI study were overweight and more hypertensive, with 40 per cent also receiving either statins or anti-hypertensive drugs, and 7.7 per cent having suffered a previous heart attack. Thus, they were not a healthy population and not at all comparable to the patients usually treated with HRT in this country. Unbelievably, they were said to have been selected for the study only if they had no symptoms.

The WHI study showed an increase in heart attacks, strokes and breast cancer, although it confirmed the decrease in colon cancer, hip fractures and spinal fractures. These complications were enough for many regulatory bodies to suggest that HRT was less safe and should be used in the lowest dose for the shortest possible time, and only for severe flushing and sweating. It was claimed that oestrogens were no longer believed to prevent heart attacks or strokes, and should not be first-line treatment for the prevention of osteoporosis.

There were not enough patients in the 50–55 age group to make any comment about the effect on heart attacks. In a subsequent WHI publication, it was clear that the increase in cardiovascular complications occurred in women over the age of 70 who started HRT. Even this population had a non-significant 11 per cent decrease in cardiovascular events if oestrogen/progestogen therapy was started within 10 years of the menopause.

One of the fundamental errors in this study is that the same dose of drug is not appropriate for all patients. The study used a combination of Premarin with continuous progestogen as a non-bleeding preparation. The epidemiologists conducting the trials were not clinicians, and were not aware that different women require different doses by different routes, or that different combinations of different hormones are needed to treat different symptoms in women of different ages. Because the Premarin/Provera combination was a totally inappropriate treatment for these older women, it was not possible to determine whether the increase in complications in older women was due to the oestrogen or the progestogen component, or a combination of both.

The oestrogen-only study was awaited with great interest. On 3 March 2003, however, it was discontinued. A midweek press conference led to the newspapers reporting that the oestrogen-only arm of the WHI study was stopped because of an increase in strokes – a claim not supported by the evidence. If we look at the patients on HRT aged 50–59, we can see there was a decrease in heart attacks of 42 per cent, a decrease in breast cancer of 28 per cent, a decrease in colon cancer of 41 per cent and a decrease in deaths of 27 per cent. There was a slight, non-significant increase in strokes of 8 per cent up to a total of 19 patients in the control group and 19 patients in the slightly larger HRT group, out of 20,000 women overall. This was hardly a reason to stop the study, which, with a few more patients, could have shown a significant decrease in the incidence of breast cancer.

There were so many faults in the design of the WHI study that I believe it will be largely discredited within another two to three years, particularly as most of the patients and most of the data from this study are inappropriate for UK practice. The study investigated a treatment we don't use on a group of patients we don't treat. The evidence that oestrogens are safe and beneficial for women below the age of 60 who have appropriate symptoms remains convincing.

Another major study that cast doubt on the safety of HRT was the Million Women's Study (MWS) from Oxford, which claimed that there was a 30 per cent increase in breast cancer in women taking unopposed oestrogens, and a greater increase in women taking oestrogen plus progestogen. The claim in this paper, that the risk begins within a year of starting HRT and disappears when it is stopped, can be criticised because of the unconvincing nature of the statistics and text. For example, of the 9,364 patients in the Million Women's Study with breast cancer, 2,224 were excluded for unexplained reasons. The peak of breast cancers detected after one year by mammography and questionnaire were most likely to have been interval cancers missed at the previous mammography, and would have had nothing to do with HRT. These cases were not excluded. There are very many other objections to the design of this study.

The usual numerical estimate of excess breast cancer that we give patients is 12 per 1,000 after 15 years of HRT. Even if this is true (and there is in fact some evidence of a *decrease* in breast cancer), it represents much the same statistical risk as that found in those taking alcohol, being overweight, having no children, having a late first pregnancy or having a late menopause.

Oestrogen treatment should be used for the treatment of specific symptoms and low bone density.

Although oestrogens appear to have no place for the secondary prevention of cardiovascular disease such as strokes and heart attacks, they may still be indicated in early symptomatic menopausal women for protection against coronary heart disease and Alzheimer's disease.

In Europe we treat young menopausal women with oestrogens. There does appear to be a window of opportunity in 45- to 60-year-old symptomatic women who may show long-term cardiovascular and neurological benefits from early oestrogen therapy. Oestrogens commenced in older 60- to 79-year-old women may cause 'early harm' in the form of heart attacks and strokes before seeing any beneficial effect upon these diseases.

The dose and route of oestrogens will depend upon the symptoms and the age of the patient. For example, women around the time of the menopause with vasomotor symptoms, such as flushes and sweats should be given oestrogen tablets or transdermal oestrogens through the skin with cyclical progestogen for protection of the uterus.

The usual duration of a progestogen course to protect the uterus is 14 days but, if the extra risk to the breast of progestogen is confirmed, it is sensible to reduce the duration of progestogen to seven days. This shortened course is also useful in women with progestogen intolerance.

Women who wish to avoid bleeding may do so by using low-dose oestrogen and progestogen, or by the use of Tibolone, or by having a Mirena IUS inserted.

Women with hormone-responsive mood disorders should have a higher dose of transdermal oestrogens by patch, gel or implant. These women are often progestogen intolerant and a seven-day cycle of progestogen is permissible.

If loss of libido and loss of energy remain a problem, the addition of testosterone should be considered.

Five-year duration of HRT has been recommended, but in reality women remain on HRT if they are feeling well and have relief of their symptoms. It is often difficult to persuade such women to discontinue treatment even after 10 or more years.

A mammogram should be performed each year and a breast examination every six months.

Chapter Twenty-five

TRANSMISSABLE SPONGIFORM ENCEPHALOPATHIES – BSE AND VCJD

BY SIR PETER LACHMANN

The Myth: BSE resulted from scientific meddling with cattle food.

The Fact: BSE arose as a rare spontaneous event and spread through the long-established, but probably ill-advised, practice of feeding cattle with 'meat and bone meal'.

The epidemic of bovine spongiform encephalopathy (BSE), or mad cow disease, that appeared without warning in the UK in the mid-1980s, and its handling by the authorities, is widely held in the media to be the main source of the British public's suspicion both of science and of government. For this reason alone, it is well worth exploring what really happened and what lessons should have been learned.

THE BACKGROUND

The original 'transmissible spongiform encephalopathy' (TSE) was scrapie, a neuro-degenerative disease of sheep that has been recognised since the eighteenth century. Affected animals itch and rub themselves against fence posts until they damage their skin, which may be the origin of the name.

In 1937, scrapie was shown to be transmissible from sheep to sheep, and later also to mice, albeit with a long incubation period. It was looked upon as a 'slow-virus' disease, without any virus having been isolated. In the 1950s, it was shown that the scrapie agent was extremely resistant to UV and to X-rays, as well as to heat and to chemical fixation. Such properties really exclude any infectious agent with a nucleic-acid genome. John Griffith, a mathematician and theoretical chemist, therefore suggested in 1967 that the scrapie agent might be a protein that can exist in two forms, one of which is infective, and that the infective form catalyses the conversion of the normal to the infectious form. This is essentially what is now regarded as the prion hypothesis.

In the 1980s, Stanley Prusiner substantially purified the scrapie agent and found it to be composed wholly of protein. He coined the term 'prion' for this protein infectious agent. It was then shown by Charles Weissmann that prions were generated from a normal protein – the prion-related protein (PrP), which was coded in the genome by a perfectly conventional gene – and that the formation of the infectious form was indeed a post-translational* event. This event involves a change in conformation (shape) involving the conversion of alpha helical structure to beta pleated sheets. The latter form becomes insoluble and very resistant to breakdown by enzymes, which forms the basis of the most commonly used test for prions. Weissmann went on to make the seminal discovery that mice with their PrP gene deleted could neither be infected with scrapie nor transmit it, showing that PrP is absolutely necessary for the disease.

The prion hypothesis is now essentially considered to be established, and its final proof – the generation of infectious prions

---

* Proteins are made in cells by, first, *transcribing* the DNA of the relevant gene into messenger RNA; and then *translating* the RNA message into protein. Subsequent changes to the protein produced by enzymes or by conformational change are called 'post-translational'.

in vitro from genetically engineered PrP – has become available in the last few months. The Nobel Committee was certainly convinced even before this, since it gave the Nobel Prize for Medicine in 1997 to Stanley Prusiner, although, with an eccentricity that is hard to fathom (although not unparalleled), it omitted Charles Weissmann.

SPONGIFORM ENCEPHALOPATHIES IN MAN

The sporadic form of spongiform encephalopathy that occurs in man is known as Creutzfeldt-Jacob disease (CJD). It affects mainly the elderly and is rapidly progressive, usually causing death in a matter of months. Its incidence is believed to be uniform worldwide at around one to two million per year. In the UK, the annual number of new cases in the last seven years has been in the range 50–74. It is significant that CJD incidence is the same in countries where scrapie in sheep is relatively common (for example, the UK) as it is in countries that are scrapie-free (such as Australia and New Zealand). This is powerful evidence against transmission of scrapie from sheep as the cause of sporadic CJD in man.

There are also rare familial forms of spongiform encephalopathy with dominant inheritance, caused by mutations in the PrP gene. These mutant forms of PrP seem to be much more prone than normal PrP to the spontaneous change in conformation that converts them to infectious prions. When brain tissue from these hereditary spongiform encephalopathies is injected into the brains of normal mice, they develop the disease which is compelling evidence against a viral cause for TSE.

There are two other important forms of human TSE. 'Kuru' is an epidemic form affecting the Fore people of New Guinea that was recognised in the 1950s. This disease was shown to be due to ritual cannibalism of brains from the dead, particularly by women and children. The epidemic seems to have started around the beginning of the twentieth century, presumably when a brain incubating sporadic CJD was eaten. The Australian authorities then forbade cannibalism and the epidemic subsided – although the last cases occurred some 50 years after the final cannibal feast. These very long incubation times occurred in people who were heterozygous (carry both forms) for a particular genetic variation in the PrP gene. All forms of human TSE are influenced by this genetic polymorphism and the heterozygotes are always the most resistant – probably because the conformational change occurs more easily if all the molecules of PrP are truly identical.

The other is 'iatrogenic' (caused by treatment) CJD. The most frequent cause was the use of human growth hormone, prepared from post-mortem human pituitary glands, to treat dwarfism. Transplantation of corneas or of brain membrane (dura mater) were rarer causes. It has been estimated that approximately 1 in 12,000 brains, apparently normal at post mortem, contain prions – and would presumably have given rise to CJD eventually. Since pools of growth hormone were made with upwards of 10,000 pituitaries it is not surprising that the pools were frequently contaminated with prions. Iatrogenic CJD is dying out, as all growth hormone used therapeutically is now genetically engineered.

The mean incubation period of iatrogenic CJD in the genetically most susceptible is in the region of seven years. This incubation period is likely to be shorter than that found when a TSE is transferred to man from another species – such as a cow – by the oral route.

BSE – BOVINE SPONGIFORM ENCEPHALOPATHY

This disease, often called mad cow disease, was first recognised in England in 1986 (although with hindsight it probably first arose in the 1970s), and rapidly assumed major epidemic proportions in the UK cattle herd. (*Figure 7* shows the number of cases diagnosed from 1986 to 2004.)

No such cattle TSE had previously been known, and the outbreak was initially confined to the United Kingdom.

The epidemiology of the outbreak was investigated by John Wilesmith at the Veterinary Laboratories Agency. He quickly came to

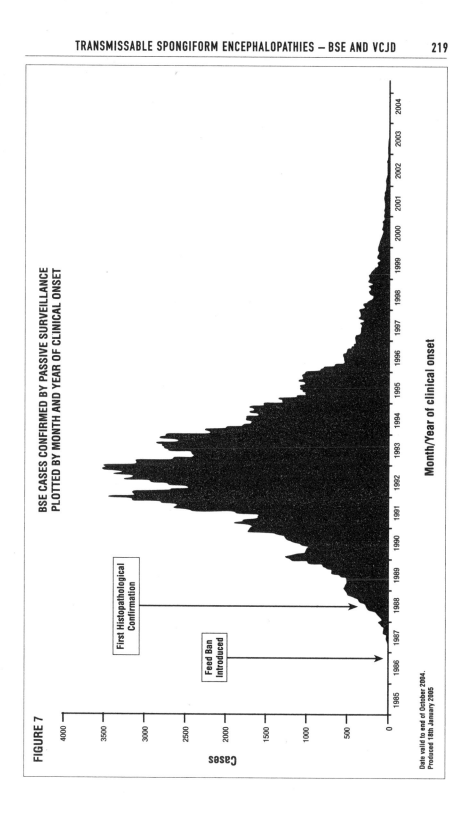

FIGURE 7

BSE CASES CONFIRMED BY PASSIVE SURVEILLANCE
PLOTTED BY MONTH AND YEAR OF CLINICAL ONSET

First Histopathological
Confirmation

Feed Ban
Introduced

Cases

Month/Year of clinical onset

Date valid to end of October 2004.
Produced 18th January 2005

the conclusion that the disease was being spread by feed and that the responsible component of the feed was 'meat and bone meal' – a product of whose existence most people were, at the time, unaware. After the obviously edible parts of an animal carcass have been removed, the rest needs to be disposed of. One of the first processes is to produce 'mechanically recovered meat' which is done by crushing the bones and harvesting the bone marrow and remaining muscle still stuck to bone, which is then processed into a cheap form of meat that can be used in sausages, pies and burgers. I shall return to this when discussing transmission of BSE to humans. What is then left is 'rendered' by heat treatment and solvent extraction, primarily to produce tallow and, as a side product, the protein-rich residue – meat and bone meal – that is added to animal feed. This has been done for much of the twentieth century all over the industrial world. In the 1970s, the process of rendering was modified. Demand for tallow was falling and the large oil-price rises of the early 1970s made the rendering process more expensive. For these reasons, the old 'batch' process (analogous to the process by which single-malt whiskey is made) was replaced by a 'continuous' process (analogous to that used in blended whiskies). This involved some lowering of the temperature at which rendering was performed. It also involved omitting the final benzene-extraction step.

Dr Wilesmith speculated that these changes may have allowed the scrapie agent in rendered sheep to survive and to infect cattle. This explanation was widely accepted at the time, but is now regarded with some scepticism. The changes in the rendering process originated in the United States and were adopted widely in the industrial world. The UK is by no means the only industrial country that has scrapie in its sheep flock, and it therefore would have been predicted that the outbreak would have occurred more widely. Furthermore, more recent, detailed inactivation studies on the BSE prion indicate that even the original rendering process fails to inactivate it. It therefore now looks highly probable that the origin of the BSE epidemic lies in the spontaneous generation of this highly unusual and very resistant form of prion in a single animal – possibly a sheep, possibly a cow, or even possibly an exotic animal like the tigers in Bristol Zoo which died of a TSE and were rendered – which entered the cattle food chain and then rapidly spread in an epidemic fashion. Such a spontaneous event must be extremely rare and the UK was very unlucky. Nevertheless, it does emphasise that it may be unwise ever to feed animals on products made from corpses of the same species. The taboo against human cannibalism may be so widespread because communities that did not adhere to it died out from TSEs!

MAVERICK EXPLANATIONS OF BSE

It was probably inevitable that a new disease with such a high economic cost and such intense media exposure should provoke denial and the increasingly familiar rash of maverick alternative theories.

The first on the scene was put forward not by a scientist but by an organic farmer, Mark Purdey, who claimed that is was phosmet, an organophosphate insecticide used to prevent warble-fly infestation, that was the real cause of BSE and that, in consequence, the disease was not spread by feed and the precautions that had been put in place were all unnecessary. It was entirely clear right from the outset that phosmet could be neither a necessary nor a sufficient cause of BSE (or any other TSE). The possibility that animals treated with phosmet might be more susceptible to prion infection was not intrinsically impossible, but no persuasive evidence for such an increased sensitivity has come to light in the intervening years. In spite of this, Mark Purdey still maintains websites(www.purdeyenvironment.com, www.markpurdey.com) giving highly idiosyncratic views on the causation not only of BSE but also now of a whole variety of other diseases.

A second, and even less convincing, hypothesis was advanced by Alan Ebringer, a professor of immunology, who proposed that BSE was an auto-immune disease due to antigenic stimulation by cross-reacting gut bacteria, and was also therefore not transmissible. The idea stemmed from a what could be a misunderstanding of experiments done by the Weissmann group. They had shown that the immune system is required for the transmission of prions from the gut to the brain, but had also shown that injection of prions directly into the brain can cause disease in fully immuno-deficient mice thereby definitively excluding that the disease is auto-immune. This has not prevented well-known journalists like William Rees-Mogg and, more recently, Magnus Linklater from defending the Ebringer view in *The Times*, not on the basis of any scientific argument, but arguing how nice it would be if the 'scientific establishment' were shown to be wrong and a maverick explanation found to be correct! This is comparable to the campaign run for many years in the *Sunday Times* defending the views of another maverick, Peter Duesberg, who suggested that AIDS is due not to HIV but to the abuse of recreational drugs.

THE GOVERNMENT RESPONSE TO THE BSE EPIDEMIC

Fortunately, there is extensive documentation on this subject from the BSE inquiry, set up by the government in December 1997 under the chairmanship of Lord Phillips. The inquiry reported in December 2000 with the Phillips Report, and is a masterpiece of its kind. The report is, however, 16 volumes long, and not many people have read it in its entirety. But it is an invaluable source of information about what went on at this time and it is still available at www.bseinquiry.gov.uk.

BSE was originally regarded purely as an animal-health problem, and it was only after some months that the chief medical officer was informed that a risk to human health should be considered. The government then set up a small working party chaired by Richard Southwood, Professor of Zoology at Oxford. The remit of the Southwood working party was to advise on the implications of BSE and matters relating thereto, and they addressed both human and animal health. They recommended at once that animals with BSE should not be allowed to enter the human food chain after slaughter, and that the carcasses be incinerated. They also recommended that the 'ruminant food ban' (already put in place by the Ministry of Agriculture) that prohibited the feeding of meat and bone meal to cattle and sheep should be made permanent. They were minded to recommend a total ban on the use of meat and bone meal, removing it altogether from the animal food chain. This recommendation was, however, not acceptable to the government on cost grounds, and in consequence it was toned down to the extent that meat and bone meal would continue to be fed to pigs and poultry, and was allowed to be exported for these purposes. This turned out to be a very bad decision, and brought to light problems in the government's advisory processes: the government expects an advisory committee to make firm recommendations, but will pressurise the committee to change recommendations if it does not like them. The Phillips Report recognised that both are defects. It is the job of expert committees to examine the scientific facts and to put forward courses of action with the benefits and risks analysed. The final decision then rests with government, which is responsible for making policy and for counting the cost. It is not acceptable for government or its civil servants to put pressure on an advisory committee to reach particular conclusions, since this subverts the advisory process. In principle, the government accepted these conclusions.

In this instance, what happened was certainly very regrettable, because, if the complete meat and bone meal ban had been implemented early in 1989, the BSE epidemic would not have taken the extreme course that it did. In practice, the partial ban proved ineffective because it turned out to be impossible adequately to separate pig and poultry food from that given to cows and sheep, and a complete ban was not put in force until 1996.

The Southwood working party favoured the scrapie origin of BSE and, taking comfort from the extensive data that scrapie does not transmit to humans, concluded that the risk to the human population was remote, although it did recommend doing research on transmission from cow to calf. Although these conclusions were justified at the time, the Phillips Report made the cogent point that, after the Southwood working party was dissolved, its recommendations were not reconsidered in the light of new information. When, in 1990, a new BSE-like disease was reported in cats and in certain zoo antelopes (which had probably had access to meat and bone meal), concerns about inter-species transmission should have been reconsidered.

There were voices warning of the dangers of BSE to man in the early 1990s. One of the more prominent was that of Professor Richard Lacey, Professor of Bacteriology at Leeds, who has a longstanding interest in food safety and infection, and who has a penchant for worst-case scenarios. He predicted that eating any beef at all was a danger and that the whole population was likely to have been contaminated (particularly from those parts of the carcass – the brain, the spinal cord and the intestine – that were known to carry prions), and predicted that there would be 2,000 cases of BSE in humans by the year 2000. This was a greatly over-pessimistic prediction, as the actual figure was 84. This and similar predictions were not based on any real data at that time.

The situation was radically transformed in 1996 when the first cases of what is now called variant CJD were described in humans by the CJD Surveillance Unit in Edinburgh. This TSE differed from the usual sporadic CJD in that it affected much younger people, had a more prolonged course and had a distinct, characteristic neuropathology. It was rapidly established that such cases were not being seen elsewhere in the world, and the conclusion was tentatively reached that this was likely to be due to the transmission of BSE to man. This was fairly rapidly confirmed, not only by the similarity of the neuropathology, but by 'strain typing' of the agent in mice. BSE seems to be a single strain of TSE, unlike scrapie where there are many strains; and the strain (as defined by neuropathology and incubation time in mice) of variant human CJD was identical to that of BSE. A biochemical method of strain typing based on glycosylation patterns of prions was introduced by Collinge, and this also demonstrated that variant CJD was identical to BSE.

At this stage, therefore, it had become clear that transmission to humans had occurred, although the scale of this was, and remains, uncertain. The possibility that a substantial epidemic of this fatal disease might occur in a relatively young population gave rise to alarm both among the public and among the regulatory authorities, and much more rigorous precautions began to be taken to exclude prions from the human food chain. The use of meat and bone meal was banned totally. This ban produced its own problems, since the disposal of meat and bone meal other than by feeding is by no means easy and it took a considerable time to achieve the necessary incineration. For long periods, meat and bone meal was stored in large amounts with the risk that rats, mice and harvest mites might be spreading it by means outside human control. Nevertheless, the complete ban on feeding meat and bone meal did bring about a further steep decline in the BSE epidemic in cattle. Perhaps surprisingly, a few new cases are still being seen about eight years after the ban was introduced, and this does raise the possibility that there may be vertical transmission from cow to calf in a rare number of instances, perhaps particularly where the cow is in the late stages of incubating the disease when the calf is born. This remains a slight problem in the final eradication of BSE from the UK herd.

There is also little doubt that the epidemic has spread widely, not only to other countries in Europe but also to most, if not all, parts of the world (see *Figure 8*), not only by the export of British cattle which may have been infected, but also by the export of meat and bone meal in the earlier years of the epidemic. Even in the last year, however, the UK still had the largest number of new cases.

VARIANT CJD

Figure 9 shows a table of all the cases of CJD referred to the surveillance unit in Edinburgh since it was set up in 1990. This

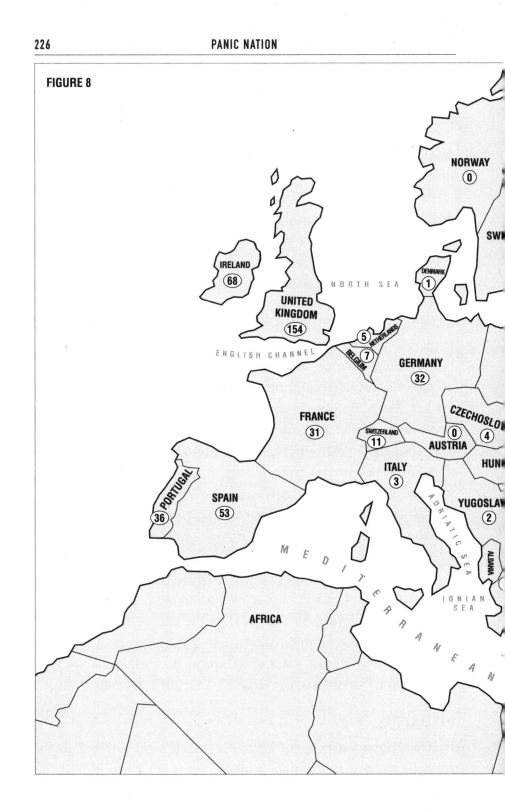

FIGURE 8

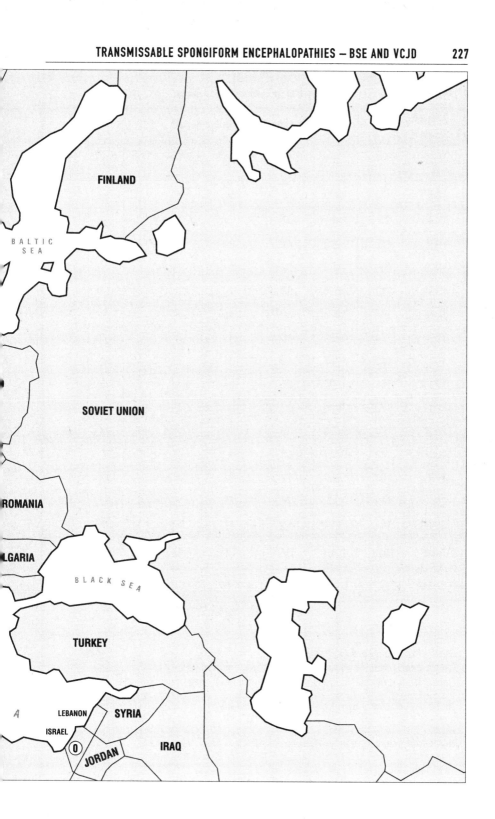

FIGURE 9   **CJD STATISTICS**

From the CJD Surveillance Unit, Edinburgh

Referrals of Suspect CJD		Deaths of definite and probable CJD						
Year	Referrals	Year	Sporadic	Iatrogenic	Familial	GSS	vCJD	Total Deaths
1990	(53)	1990	28	5	0	0	-	33
1991	75	1991	32	1	3	0	-	36
1992	96	1992	45	2	5	1	-	53
1993	78	1993	37	4	5	2	-	46
1994	118	1994	53	1	4	3	-	61
1995	87	1995	35	4	2	3	3	47
1996	134	1996	40	4	2	4	10	60
1997	161	1997	60	6	4	1	10	81
1998	154	1998	63	3	3	2	18	89
1999	170	1999	62	6	2	0	15	85
2000	178	2000	50	1	2	1	28	82
2001	179	2001	58	4	3	2	20	87
2002	163	2002	72	0	4	1	17	94
2003	162	2003	76	5	4	2	18	105
2004	112	2004	46	1	2	1	9	59
Total Referrals	**1920**	**Total Deaths**	**757**	**47**	**43**	**23**	**148**	**1018**

SUMMARY OF VCJD CASES

Deaths
Deaths from definite vCJD (confirmed):   106
Deaths from probable vCJD (without neuropathological confirmation):   41
Deaths from probable vCJD (neuropathological confirmation pending):   1

Number of deaths from definite or probable vCJD: 148

Alive
Number of definite/probable vCJD cases still alive: 5

Total number of definite or probable vCJD cases (dead and alive):   153

shows not only the sporadic disease but also the other forms. It can be seen that by the end of December 1994 the total number of definite vCJD cases was 152. The annual number of cases started at around 10 per year, rose to a maximum (so far) of 28 in 2000, and since then has, if anything, slightly declined. The interpretation of these figures is not entirely clear because there is no accurate information on the average incubation period and because it is not known when the human population was first exposed to the agent. Those so far showing disease may have genetically determined high susceptibility and short incubation periods, or may have been exposed to unusually large amounts of the agent early in the outbreak. However, the time of maximum exposure to infection from infected beef products was probably between 1990 and 1992. This was about 14 years ago, and it is becoming possible to be reasonably hopeful that the annual number of cases (from this source) will not increase dramatically in the future. However, it is highly likely that new cases will continue to appear for several decades.

HOW DID HUMANS GET INFECTED?

The finger of suspicion has been pointed at mechanically recovered meat as the most likely source of prions in the human food chain. This has been used in the manufacture of cheap burgers, sausages and meat pies, and may have been eaten particularly by children. The use of mechanically recovered meat from cattle was banned in 1995 and the use of all 'specified bovine offal' in human food had been forbidden since 1989, so the chance of food-borne infection in the UK must now be remote. One small cluster of cases was attributed to poor slaughter practices by a local butcher.

The extent of human-to-human spread by blood transfusion or tissue transplantation is difficult to predict, although so far there are only one or two authenticated cases and precautions have been put in place.

WHAT IS NEEDED NOW?

There is now an urgent need to develop tests for prions that are sufficiently sensitive to detect infection in the blood early in the incubation period. Only when this is achieved will it be possible to make accurate estimates of the number of people (and animals) carrying the infection, and to make accurate predictions of the future extent of the epidemic. Such a test would also be invaluable for screening blood and tissue donors.

Furthermore, when treatments are developed – and a number of agents that interfere with the conversion of PrP to prions are under study – one can be fairly confident that they will be effective mainly, or only, in the pre-clinical phase of the disease. By the time that symptoms appear there is already substantial destruction of brain tissue from which recovery will be difficult.

CONCLUSIONS

BSE was a disaster for the livestock industry and hugely expensive for the whole country. Variant CJD is a lethal disease of young people, which is a tragedy, but, unless there are very unpleasant surprises to come, its scale is likely to be limited and not to be compared, even in the UK, with the tragedy of AIDS. It is to be expected that cases will continue to occur for several decades but there is every reason to hope that the number of new cases will not rise appreciably above the current level of approximately 20 per year. The dire predictions made, largely in the lay media, soon after the recognition of vCJD have not come about.

The BSE epidemic arose from a rare spontaneous event and became an epidemic as a result of feeding cattle with products made from cattle carcasses, a practice that had been used throughout the industrialised world for many decades but is now banned. The outbreak was not due, contrary to much media opinion, to any novel science being introduced into animal husbandry. The government response had faults in the early stages, not least in its public utterances, but the cattle epidemic has been brought under control.

The mavericks added nothing of value and the media, on the whole, have little to congratulate themselves about. The scientists involved in prion research, on the other hand, have less with which to reproach themselves.

Chapter Twenty-six

ARE WE BEING POISONED BY THE AIR WE BREATHE?

BY JOHN HENRY

The Myth: Pollutants in the air are seriously harmful to health.

The Fact: The air is cleaner and healthier than it has been for at least 100 years.

Are we being poisoned by the air we breathe? This is a frightening thought – the purity of the air we breathe is one of the aspects of our lives that as individuals we have very little control over. Because of this, air pollution has been a major concern among environmentalists and citizens for many years. However, I hope this article will help you to conclude that the overall news is good.

Let us start by looking back in time, in order to see if we can find a baseline. History books tell us that the air in our cities has been polluted for millennia. Even ancient Rome used to have an air-pollution problem. Fifty years ago in Britain, most of the public buildings in our cities used to be black, covered with sooty deposits from atmospheric pollution. However, once the air quality was improved, the buildings were all cleaned up. Now, on any sunny day it can be clearly seen that the glistening white stone remains clean to the present. Older people will still remember the atmospheric pollution and 'smog' – a combination of smoke and fog – that used to be a frequent occurrence in many cities in Britain. As a boy in southeast London I well remember the 1950s when the smog outbreaks occurred. I recall my father, a general practitioner, coming home with black soot around his nostrils and giving our family the list of people we knew in the neighbourhood who had died that day. It was incidents like these that led to the improvements in air quality from which we now benefit. Many potential pollutants have been reduced or eliminated. Lead from petrol, asbestos particles, industrial, vehicle and domestic emissions have all been reduced thanks to the introduction of smokeless fuels and processes that reduce or prevent the escape of particles into the atmosphere. All of this provides us with evidence that air quality has changed in the developed countries, and I would suggest markedly for the better, over the last half-century and longer.

So are we being poisoned by the air we breathe, or are we being scared by the way that stories are being presented? It is the role of the press to supply us with facts; but nowadays it seems they have to be stark and unusual enough to produce the headlines that sell a newspaper. For example, we often see news articles about the risks of passive smoking, which upsets and concerns many people. But there are far fewer articles about the dangers of smoking, which is a very much greater hazard. And the result is that many people seem to be equally concerned about passive smoking as about tobacco smoking itself, without realising what a massive difference there is between the two!

Particles in the air are known to be a major cause of long-term respiratory illness. Miners used to suffer from pneumoconiosis due to breathing the particles of coal dust in mines. Overall, less than 10 per cent of particles in the air are man-made, so the vast majority do *not* come from combustion or machinery, but the proportion in cities tends to be higher. In recent years, there has been much talk about inorganic particles in the atmosphere being linked to death from a number of medical conditions. And it is clear that this is a real effect

– it is possible to track all the hospital admissions and deaths occurring in a locality and to compare them with the data about the mass concentrations of PM_{10} or $PM_{2.5}$ (milligrams of particulate matter less than 10 m or 2.5 m aerodynamic diameter per cubic metre) in the air day by day. There are more hospital admissions and deaths on the days when there is more PM in the air. But the increase in deaths is small, and they tend to occur in people who are already ill. The overall effect is that people may be admitted to hospital when PM levels are high, and some may die a few days earlier or later than they would have otherwise done, depending on the amount of PM in the air.

This, at least, was believed until very recently. The latest statistical methods show that the lag between a change in particle levels and increased daily deaths may extend from a day to more than a month. However, it is unlikely that healthy people are much affected by daily fluctuations in levels of air pollution. Long-term exposure to fine particles ($PM_{2.5}$) is thought to be associated with an increased risk of dying from cardiovascular disease. The evidence shows that, after personal factors such as smoking, occupation and diet have been allowed for, there remains an association between long-term levels of particles and the risk of dying from cardiovascular disease. This was clearly demonstrated some years ago: a distinct drop in the death rate from cardiovascular disease followed the banning of all coal sales in Dublin. Clearly, there is a need to further reduce the numbers of particles in the atmosphere, but any effect of reducing peak levels will not be dramatic.

Despite intensive research, there is very little evidence on whether any one type of particle is at fault – it appears that the size of particle is the most important factor. Current thinking suggests that the smallest particles in the air may play an important role. These particles (nanoparticles) occur in large numbers but contribute little to mass concentrations expressed as PM_{10} or $PM_{2.5}$. It has been suggested that these tiny particles set up an inflammatory response in the lung which, by a complex chain of consequences, causes atherosclerotic lesions in the coronary arteries to become unstable. Evidence in support of this theory is accumulating, and we are likely to hear more about the illnesses caused by nanoparticles in the air.

Another topic that often finds its way into the news is the number of people who suffer from, and who die from, asthma. Asthma is increasing in frequency, especially among young people, and asthma-related deaths are also on the increase. This is a fact, but it is unlikely to be due to pollution in the air – if anything, it is the reverse! Asthma is now believed to have become more common because people live in much cleaner environments, so that they are not exposed to allergens such as house dust mites when they are very small children. This means that the body does not come to consider these foreign proteins as part of its 'normal' environment and, when children eventually do come in contact with them at a later stage, the body reacts by developing an allergy to them. So the most developed theory to explain the increase in asthma is that small children are not exposed to pollutants at the point in their development when they would treat them as normal components of their environment. However, combustion from domestic fires and motor vehicles produces oxides of nitrogen and other chemical substances that can worsen asthma. There is, therefore, a clear link between atmospheric pollution by the products of combustion and the severity of asthma, so asthma can be worse when combustion is common and when the wind and weather conditions are unfavourable.

Another question that is asked about asthma is its relationship to thunderstorms. What environmental factor is involved here? There is an increase in severe asthma after thunderstorms, and this is because under normal conditions pollen particles are not able to reach the small airways and their effect is limited. But in the very humid air after a thunderstorm, pollen particles break open, releasing the protein particles within. These particles are breathed in and pass much further down the air passages, triggering asthma.

So the conclusion is that there are many factors in the air that are linked with illness, but atmospheric pollution is decreasing due to the concerted efforts of many governments, universities and industrial concerns, and the air is safer to breathe than it has been for many years. This does not mean that we should be complacent, but it is encouraging.

Chapter Twenty-seven

REPETITIVE STRAIN INJURY

BY PAUL AICHROTH

The Myth: Repetitive Strain Injury is a serious health risk deriving from our modern lifestyle.

The Fact: Much RSI is due to the compensation culture; genuine cases can be very successfully treated.

Nearly all of us has suffered from a repetitive strain, whether it was caused by a vigorous game of tennis, writing a thesis longhand, typing on an old-fashioned mechanical typewriter or opening too many bottles of wine at a Christmas party. The ache is closely associated with any movement similar to that causing the strain in the first place. It usually gets better after a few hours' or days' rest, avoiding using the painful muscle or tendon. Very occasionally, when the pain persists and the area becomes sensitive and swollen, we talk of the condition as a 'repetitive strain injury' (RSI).

RSI, as its name implies, is caused by a stress or physical force which has been repeatedly applied in the same way. Unlike the simple 'sprain', it does not get better within a day or two, indeed in some cases it may persist for months. Although there is no doubt that it is the strain that causes the condition, there is also a personal, idiosyncratic element in determining the severity of the pain produced, which differs from one individual to another. It is highly unpredictable: some people exposed to exactly the same conditions over the same period will fail to develop the painful inflammation characteristic of RSI; others find that the pain that develops is out of keeping with the physical evidence of inflammation. This makes it very difficult, in most industrial circumstances, to take precautions to prevent it from happening.

The implications of RSI are economic and legal as well as medical. The US Bureau of Statistics estimates that there are 70,000 cases in the USA each year and the number is increasing. Each case costs between $7,000 and $30,000, and the total expense approaches $200 million a year. In addition, each case causes an average of 18 days' absence from work.

The medico-legal implications are considerable: although the cause may appear obvious, liability is often difficult to assess. Even the diagnosis may be controversial. Where swelling and inflammation is apparent, or an X-ray shows a stress fracture of a bone, the diagnosis is clear, but in a substantial number of cases the pain described is out of proportion to the tissue damage or no inflammation can be detected. Compensationitis, a symptom without an apparent physical cause that is often protracted but usually disappears once a claim for compensation is agreed, undoubtedly accounts for a number of these cases. In others, a psychological dysfunction such as anxiety or depression may underlie the condition. There is little doubt that an increasing number of the complaints of RSI are motivated by a wish to obtain time off work or other financial benefit. Because of the suspicion that many cases of those claiming to be victims of repetitive strain injury are manipulative, it is important to be able to separate the genuine injuries from the bogus ones, and to be able to assess the degree to which the individual patient's particular susceptibility, rather than the strain to which he or she was exposed, was responsible for the condition.

THE DIAGNOSIS

There are certain parts of the body that are regularly stressed and strained during specific activities and exercises. Usually these areas take the stress easily without pain or ill effects. However, in some patients a repetitive strain in the same part of the body produces inflammation, a tearing of soft tissues and occasionally a bone fracture. The anatomical structures affected by repetitive strains and injuries are:

Tendons
Muscles
Musculo-tendinous junctions
Tendon insertions into bone
Bone

Tendons

The tendons in the hand and wrist are commonly affected. A repetitive strain from using a computer, typing or writing can inflame the tendon sheath. Each of the tendons in the hand and wrist run in a sheath which is lubricated by a small amount of fluid. If the movements are repetitive, and especially if they are forced, the sheath may become inflamed and swollen, producing pain and swelling. There is local tenderness and sometimes a creaking sensation. The inflammation is called tenosynovitis. The condition is very painful and any movement of the finger or wrist aggravates the situation. The patient usually needs to take time off work. The treatment is to rest the inflamed tendon and to splint the fingers or the wrist and give anti-inflammatory medication. If the problem recurs then a local injection of hydrocortisone, together with local anaesthetic, often speeds up recovery.

Muscles

The muscles of the upper limb are prone to RSI. This is frequently seen in musicians. Pain, swelling and tenderness may result from the repetitive movement which is part of the musician's normal activity. It is treated with immediate rest; in some situations splinting the area may be necessary in order to rest it. The tender area of muscle can be treated by the physiotherapist using massage, muscle stretching and local ultrasound.

The repetitive nature of the musician's activity frequently produces a recurrence and the treatment may have to be repeated time and again. It is not uncommon for a musician whose performance is deteriorating to use the symptoms and the diagnosis as an excuse or as a means of obtaining compensation, redundancy or sympathy.

Musculo-tendinous Junctions

The junction between the large calf musculature and the top of the Achilles tendon is especially prone to repetitive strains in runners and joggers. A partial rupture is sometimes seen in jumpers, tennis players and skiers. The same principles of diagnosis and treatment apply, but in this situation the use of an injection of hydrocortisone is not recommended as it weakens the fibrous tissue of the upper tendon and makes it susceptible to full rupture. A raised heel in the shoe is useful, and with the help of a physiotherapist a successful outcome is usual, but it may take a long time.

Tendon Insertions into Bone

Tennis elbow is extremely painful and may be due to the repetitive strains of tennis. If tennis is the main cause, it is usually down to excessive backhand strokes. When the forearm is extended, the muscles are strained at their fibrous attachment to the outside of the end of the humerus, at the elbow. The muscles that bend the elbow, the flexors, are attached at the inside of the end of the humerus. Pain at this spot is usually referred to as 'golfer's elbow'. After initial rest, possibly using a sling, the inflammation usually settles. In a few patients the condition goes on to become chronic. In this situation, a strap applied just below the elbow often helps. Again, an injection of hydrocortisone and local anaesthetic seems to cure some 50 per cent of the cases. It may have to be repeated two to three times.

Bone

Repeated activity associated with extension of the knee in children aged between 10 and 13, such as jumping and kicking, may tear a small particle of bone from the immature upper end of the tibia where the tendon from the kneecap meets the bone. A small separate bone, an ossicle, may be seen on X-ray. In this condition the area around the upper end of the tibia is excessively painful and tender. The condition usually cures itself over many months, during which time sports will have to be curtailed. Although it is unlikely to lead to a claim for compensation, it may be a reason for getting out of school.

New army recruits who are subjected to repeated marching classically injure the small bones in their feet. Immediate diagnosis of a fracture may be difficult as the X-ray changes are often not apparent initially, but a bone scan will always show them.

Running may injure the tibia, especially when carrying heavy packs. This is the cause of a serious stress fracture. Treatment may require immobilisation using a plaster cast. I saw a group of 15 officer cadets – all very fit young men in their late teens who were subjected to enormous physical efforts, such as running while carrying telegraph poles! Four of this group developed stress fractures to the foot or the tibia. This type of excessive training borders on physical abuse. Training to this excessive degree is counter-productive – in these recruits it interrupted their training for many months. These highly motivated and loyal young men never took any compensatory action.

There is little doubt that, although repetitive strain injury does occur, the number claiming to be victims of the condition is inflated by those hoping to benefit from being labelled as sufferers of RSI. The question of liability is a legal minefield. In the case of the soldiers subjected to unreasonable stress, the injuries were clearly due to unnecessary trauma; but when someone develops a painful tenosynovitis of the wrist after opening bottles of wine at a friend's party, they can hardly expect that the friend should be legally liable for their pain and suffering. Between these two extremes lies a fertile field for the lawyers. It is made more complicated by the difficulty in distinguishing between those suffering from an obvious case of repetitive strain injury and those in whom the pain and distress is out of proportion to the physical evidence of tissue damage and in whom the diagnosis can never be entirely satisfactory.

Chapter Twenty-eight

THE NEW SPORT OF TESTING FOR SPORTS DRUGS

BY SAM SHUSTER

The Myth: Drug–taking by a few is the scourge of the sporting world.

The Fact: Taking drugs for sport performance and training is very common; this is no more 'unfair' than other training methods and there is no proof drugs improve performance.

Before the Athens Olympics, I was hoping that at least half the main participant teams would be caught out by positive drug tests. This is not because I believe these teams take more drugs than others – let's not fool ourselves, drug-taking by athletes and sportsmen and women is pretty well universal. No, my reason was much more pragmatic: the banning and withdrawal of such a large number of participants would have effectively closed the games and that would not have been tolerated. It would have killed off for all time the aggressive and oppressive stupidity of testing for 'performance-enhancing drugs' – a stupidity that has spoiled many sports events, and led to the banning of many good, honest athletes and the destruction of their careers. In the event, too few of the drug-takers were caught to reveal the absurdity of drug-testing, and the games began with the banning of two very popular Greek champions.

The new sport of baiting athletes and sportspeople by testing for performance-enhancing drugs is becoming sport's equivalent of the Inquisition. The philosophical belief is that the competition can only be 'fair' if performed in accordance with what certain people believe to be fair. This meaningless circular argument inevitably excludes drugs believed to be performance promoters, and leads to the creation of a drug-testing 'industry' with its panel of invasive inquisitors. This industry started with the opportunistic, but innocent, use of drugs in sport, and came to its thoughtless, lumbering climax with the development of special techniques for their detection. The underlying assumptions to this development are:

1. Certain drugs are effective as performance promoters.
2. Taking them is ethically wrong.

I believe both of these assumptions are questionable.

For the participant, sport has two main objectives: the enjoyment of participation and the desire to win – which includes the personal, social and financial consequences that may follow. Drug usage is widespread in recreational sports. The drugs are taken in the hope of seeing an improvement in performance or a greater enjoyment in participation. Apart from the inevitable and generally ignored warnings about drug risks, nobody seems to be greatly concerned about this usage of drugs in sport. This is in contrast to the opprobrium and coercive testing when drugs are taken in competitive sports. The reasons given for this, which are assumed to be self-evidently correct, are the crude, closed-minded notions of preventing 'cheating' and maintaining 'fairness', hidden by the well-muddied cliché of a 'level playing field'. But do these worn-out verbal blankets really apply to athletics? Connecting up a false alarm to your epée, or concealed running in a walking race (or perhaps more amusingly, hitching a lift) is cheating, because it gains marks that don't belong to that activity. But what of performance-enhancing drugs? They do not gain marks other than for performance in the activity being undertaken. If, after taking a drug, you fence to a win, it is for a proper strike, not a fake electrical one. It isn't a cheated victory just because it's a drug-aided one.

So what, then, is wrong with being helped by drugs? Surely, if it is acceptable to improve your skill and performance by training, then why not by drugs? If you know your competitor has better staying power in a sport that needs staying power, why is it acceptable to go away and train to build up your staying power, so long as you don't use drugs? The main objection seems to be to the use of materials other than those naturally accessible to the individual sportsman – an idea, born long ago, of a pure, individual effort. This would mean no crampons, ropes or oxygen for climbing, and no special hulls for sailboats. And what of the use of specialised training equipment? How natural are those carefully monitored gymnasia, with equipment and facilities well outside the range and pockets of most people – even, sometimes, to other competing athletes and sportspeople? And how can we reject drugs when we accept that our star athletes are wired up to highly specialised electronic equipment, in semi-secret laboratories skilled in monitoring physiological activities of heart, nerve, muscle and brain in order to provide information that is then used to maximise the athlete's performance?

Or again, on a simpler but no less important level, what of the use of skilled professional sports trainers to maximise physical performance, and coaching by sports psychologists to 'sharpen' (I hesitate to use the word 'improve') the mental activity and characteristics essential to high-level sports performance? Why is the use of a team of professional sports 'performance enhancers', from doctors, physiotherapists, dietitians and psychologists to equipment specialists (who replace a swimmer's skin with an artificial cover giving better aqua-dynamic properties) more acceptable than a few pills? What is more fair, a pill or a Schumacher-sized team of 'assistants'? And why is tampering with major constituents of the diet acceptable, when dietary modification can have just as profound a pharmacological effect as a drug – it can even replace drugs in the treatment of diseases such as diabetes. What, other than out-dated and irrational bias, is the objection to using haemopoietin injections to increase red blood cell mass (thought to give more the body more oxygen per puff), but not to training at altitude, which does the same thing? Haemopoietin injections might be more readily available to Dutch athletes than the more expensive option of travelling to train at altitude. If anything, therefore, it can be argued that performance-enhancing drugs would allow greater equality of access: they could create the level playing field so beloved by politicians and others who run short of justification for their case.

Inconsistency is the clue to irrationality. A simple illustration of this is the tolerant attitude of the sportsdrugophobes to the strips of adhesive plaster many footballers and runners now sport on the nose. Let's, for the moment, assume the dubious to be correct – that they increase oxygenation: why is this acceptable, when a drug, which achieves the same objective by decreasing lung airway resistance, is not? Just because the plaster is external and inert doesn't obviate its purpose. Otherwise, if being external and inert makes a performance enhancer acceptable, would that not justify the use of an arm extension by a short basketball player? What is and isn't considered 'cheating' is arbitrary; and, as we have already seen, the case against sports drug usage is consistently inconsistent, as befits its irrationality.

The maintenance of 'fairness' is the other argument made by the anti-drug sports fanatics.

Fairness in sport? They've got to be joking! Competitive sport is all about doing better, if not being better, than your competitor. Does it matter that basketball is played by giants whose main problem is reaching *down* to the basket? Shouldn't 'fairness' insist that basketball be played in leagues in which players are graded by the centimetre? And what about the biological unfairness of possessing a quicker tactical wit? We are in danger of confusing equality with fairness: wouldn't the rational extension of the argument used to ban drugs (to ensure 'fairness') be the inspection of sportspeople to determine their equality? And wouldn't we need to be sure that they were not, for example, doing more than a permitted training stint each day (agreed upon, of course, by an inspecting committee) to exclude any unfair advantage. Perhaps, in place of drug-testing, we could have a sports-training inspector.

Fairness in competitive sport? The whole venture is about gaining an advantage, and there is no difference between accepting those happily conferred by a sporty gene, and those gained by training and assistance, including the use of drugs. Indeed, it could be argued that, by flattening out differences between individuals, drugs could make sports competition more 'fair'. It has been argued that the reason drug-taking is cheating is that it is done covertly. But most of the acceptable things athletes do are covert: if a runner found a training method that improved the speed of their start, they would certainly not pass it on to competitors. Distance runners study their opponents and conceal their plan about when to kick for home. And in any case, if the covert nature of taking drugs for sport is the real objection, the solution is simple: make it open and free to all

What of the drugs themselves? The underlying assumption in the case against drugs in sport is that they augment performance by a purely pharmacological effect, yet, by using the standard, conventional criteria for acceptance of a drug for clinical use, there are no studies to show that sports drugs actually work: absolutely none! It may surprise those who so vociferously oppose drug usage in sport, but there have never been any acceptable, double-blind, randomised, placebo-controlled studies (such as are absolutely essential before any drug can be considered effective for a clinical purpose) showing that any 'performance-enhancing drug' actually improves an actual athletic or sporting performance. That is not to say that some of the drugs used may not work, but that there is no acceptable evidence that they do.

What has led to the use of drugs in sport is a perversion of current clinical and pharmacological practice. Sportsmen are always aiming to go one better than their competitors – that is the nature of the game – and their trainers and coaches are constantly on the lookout for ways of doing this. Many drugs in general use have been found to have discrete effects in laboratory studies, and it has been assumed that these effects would be translated to real-life situations, other than in the treatment of disease. But, of course, life is more complex than that, and many drugs in therapeutic use have overall effects quite unlike the properties for which they were introduced. Haemopoietin is the exception and, despite the absence of clinical trials involving sports activities, it is reasonable to suppose the end result will mimic altitude training. With most of the other drugs used in sport, the extrapolative assumptions in making the run from lab to lap are far less certain. For example, androgens – male hormones, and the most commonly used drugs in sport – will increase muscle bulk; but this is no reason for assuming this will lead to an increase in the performance of a 100-metre race, or facilitate the production of an ace tennis serve, let alone the skills of a star footballer. And indeed there is no evidence of such an effect, despite the banning of the drug together with the sad athletes caught taking them.

The enormous list of banned drugs is matched only by the enormity of the assumptions used to justify banning them. The argument that, because of the special rewards now consequent on winning, banning of drugs is needed is specious. There is a lack of proof of the efficacy of the drugs concerned in conferring an advantage, and the testing only reveals a small proportion of the many who may take the drugs. Finally, whereas the beneficial effects are unproven, their harmful effects are well established.

But this is no more reason for drug-testing in sportspeople than testing for the covert ingestion of hamburgers in the obese.

So far, we've considered the case for the banning of sports drugs; now let's consider the case against such a banning.

Ask any sportsperson and they will tell you that most competitive and many recreational athletes and sportspeople take drugs; but, as we all know, only a small proportion are caught. Now, if taking drugs is unfair and most competing sportspeople take them, isn't it even more unfair if only a proportion is going to be punished? As well as being unfair to sportspeople, the careers of many have been permanently blighted by them being found out and banned for life.

Athletes and sportspeople in their prime are being cast aside, with all the personal, social and financial consequences that it entails, at a time when colleagues, who are also taking the drugs, continue because they've not been found out. Think of the sadness that must have led to the two Greek heroes' motorcycle 'accident'. The penalty given to the offending sportspeople is far too great; it is out of all proportion to the 'crime'.

Even more troubling is the ever-expanding sports-drug-testing industry, and its persecuting zeal, reliant as it is for its own livelihood on the very drug-taking it affects to wish to destroy. But, as nature has shown, good parasites know they must never kill their host. So, although the drug-testing industry and its panel of inquisitors will keep on expanding, producing and using ever more invasive tests (top athletes can't even pee in private) and wasting more money and manpower on an unnecessary technology, it knows that the athletes will stay ahead. After all, that is what they are trained to do: they'll continue to find newer, still undetectable drugs, as well as new ways of disguising what they have already taken.

Sadly, instead of a relaxed discussion, the problem has been magnified and worsened by its reporting in the media. Sport has been devalued and unbalanced by the good copy to be made from horror stories about drug-taking. One effect of these reports in the media is that the testing of athletes and sportspeople for drugs is itself becoming a sport.

The effect created by the media's uncritical magnification of the sports-drug story has been unhelpful and has upset sport's followers as well as its practitioners. Most of those who enjoy watching sport are more concerned with seeing a good game than worrying about how the players achieve it. The media has not put a full, balanced case for public consideration. Many opportunities have been missed, and the presentation of a worthwhile, informed discussion has been eclipsed by the usual horror stories. Most people I've spoken to want good sport; they don't want the disturbances and disappointments that come from drug-testing. What would the people really think if the weakness of the case against sports drugs was presented without the emotive language about cheats and national shame? Perhaps, despite the bad press and negligible discussion, the public has already guessed that sports-drug-testing does not make sense.

There is no proof that drugs improve sporting activity, and even if they did it would be no more unfair than the well-accepted special training programmes. It is time we stopped restricting the use of drugs in sport, along with the sport of baiting sportspeople. It's up to the participants to decide for themselves what they want and need to do to further their sports performance. It's none of our business: it's their choice for their activity. Whose sport is it anyway?

Chapter Twenty-nine

COMPLEMENTARY MEDICINE: INTEGRATED WAFFLE?

BY MICHAEL FITZPATRICK

The Myth: Complementary medicine can be as effective as orthodox medicine.

The Fact: There is little scientific evidence to suggest that complementary medicine is at all effective.

One of the worst things that could happen in the NHS would be the double standard of the introduction of unscientific, opinion-based therapies to 'complement' or replace evidence based on orthodox medicine. Unfortunately, this is precisely what the waffle about 'integrated medicine' seems to be all about. It is in danger of taking us back to the Dark Ages by advocating a form of political correctness in order to appease powerful pressure groups.

Edzard Ernst, Britain's first professor of complementary medicine, condemned New Labour's plans to instruct Britain's GPs to refer patients to practitioners of the various diverse arts of complementary medicine which were introduced as part of the wider campaign to integrate unproven complementary practices into primary-care medicine within the NHS. This campaign has won the enthusiastic sponsorship of Prince Charles and the endorsement of the former radical activist Peter Hain, now Secretary of State for Northern Ireland and Wales.

The advocacy of alternative medicine by the Prince of Wales is consistent with his heritage. The conservative, aristocratic tradition has been reluctant to come to terms with the changes wrought by the Enlightenment and the French Revolution that brought great social and political changes as a consequence of an attempt to organise society according to principles based on reason. Those who have sought to turn back the wheel of history have upheld the principles of divine and ecclesiastical authority, tradition and social hierarchy. Over the past century, these reactionaries and their followers have provided the natural base for conservationist and environmentalist causes. They have also patronised and promoted mystical cults such as theosophy, and alternative healing systems such as homeopathy. One of the curiosities of the past 30 years is that many of these views have been taken up by middle-class activists and disillusioned radicals, like Peter Hain, who have played a key role in giving them the legitimacy and mainstream popularity they have recently come to enjoy.

The pursuit of reason and truth is central to the advance of civilisation, and hostility to science is inherently regressive. It is expressed in the tendency to suppress all notions of scientific and technological innovation, while espousing mystical conceptions of nature, the cosmos and personal spirituality. Such views are now commonly embraced by post-modernist cynics as well as by the traditional conservatives. A common feature of this trend is the emphasis given to immediate thoughts, feelings and sensations, and a neglect of the importance of reflection and new theories in the development of ideas. This anti-humanist tendency fuses the interactions between humanity, nature, the individual and society into a single unit: from their perspective, humans and nature are at one and never in conflict. Whatever is natural must therefore be good for man. This approach results in degrading the importance of individuality and rationality.

The trend for packaging us as a metaphysical unit results in the abandonment of the historic concept of Cartesian dualism (the radical separation of mind and body declared by the French philosopher Rene Descartes in the seventeenth century) by the world of complementary health. According to Deepak Chopra, renegade endocrinologist and leading alternative-health guru, 'The body is not a mindless machine; the body and mind are one.' Candace Pert, a neuroscientist who has embraced what she characterises as the 'new paradigm', favours the term 'bodymind' to express the way that 'the brain is integrated into the body at a molecular level'. For Pert, the bodymind is part of the 'unity of life' resulting from the ubiquitous polypeptides that act as transmitters in all forms of animal life: 'Humans share a common heritage, the molecules of emotion, with the most modest of microscopic creatures.'

But what is achieved by replacing Descartes's concept of mechanically opposed mind and body with a metaphysically (and terminologically) unified bodymind? The central problem highlighted by Descartes, that of discovering the relationship between the mind and the body, is replaced by a vacuous holism by these advocates of holistic therapies. Whereas Descartes's approach was a historic innovation that provided the basis for modern medical science, the concept of bodymind is a retreat from science into mysticism. Pert's notion of the 'mobile brain' – what she characterises as 'an apt description of the psychosomatic network through which intelligent information travels from one system to another' is as unlikely as the nineteenth-century notion of the mobile uterus, which was believed to travel around the female body producing hysterical symptoms. It is no surprise to discover that, having turned her back on science, Pert has become an advocate of New Age mysticism and alternative healing.

The key challenge to scientific medicine is to explain the pathological processes that are the cause of disease states, and to deal with the experience of illness. In dealing with the reality of human disease, reason, despite all its limitations, is the best weapon we've got. Reason tells us that medical science has proved to be dramatically effective in the treatment of a wide range of diseases, from infections to endocrine disorders, in which the pathological processes are fairly well understood. The success of modern scientific medicine is the principal reason why it has prevailed over diverse ancient alternatives (many of which have now re-emerged under the complementary-health umbrella). In other conditions, such as coronary heart disease and cancer, major killers of our time, where our medical understanding is less complete and therapy less effective, it is possible to assess the benefits of different treatments and to measure their adverse effects. The judgement of the value of any particular treatment is made with reference to a body of scientific knowledge which is, at least in theory and increasingly in practice, available to the patient as well as to the doctor. (By contrast, the client of the alternative practitioner has to rely on faith alone.)

In some conditions, such as multiple sclerosis or motor-neurone disease, medical understanding remains limited and treatment virtually non-existent. In these conditions the patients are in a situation similar to that which prevailed in relation to most diseases a century ago. Yet, just as most patients with multiple sclerosis today opt for conventional rather than alternative medicine, so patients in the past put their trust in scientific medicine. Why they chose orthodox medicine rather than the diverse alternatives on offer before medical science first began to yield effective treatments has long been a matter of controversy among historians. Some have attributed the success of orthodox medicine to the political and organisational skills of the early medical professionals. A more likely explanation is that the commitment of doctors to the advance of medical science persuaded most patients that it was more likely to be beneficial than the mystical alternatives on offer.

Writing in 1859, the German physician Bernard Naunyn observed that doctors' zeal won patients' respect and trust: 'It never occurred to them to inquire whether this zeal was in the interest of treatment or in the interest of science.' At a time when all treatment was experimental, patients and doctors joined in a collective endeavour against disease. Even in these cynical times, most patients still uphold this rational spirit – only to find some doctors retreating from it.

There has been greater criticism of the record of scientific medicine and the medical profession in dealing with the subjective experience of illness. Yet this criticism neglects the major advances that have occurred in recent years. In the heyday of scientific medicine, from the 1940s to the 1960s, doctors seemed to take little interest in the emotional and psychological aspects of their patients' illnesses. The emergence of scientific medicine, as a replacement for the older traditional systems of healing, caused the modern practitioners to distance themselves from an evangelical and charismatic style of practice. The quest for rational therapeutic regimes was associated with a conscious drive to eschew the less rational aspects of medical practice. Once doctors were in a position to prescribe effective drugs – and to replace hips and carry out kidney transplants and open-heart surgery – they came to rely less on a good bedside manner. Traditional 'physicianly' skills were allowed to lapse to a point where some doctors, especially in surgical specialities, seemed inclined to dispense even with elementary civilities.

The bureaucratisation of medical practice, whether through systems of insurance or state welfare, helped to make doctors less and less personally involved with the pain and suffering of their patients. The persistence of these trends towards a more mechanistic and algorithmic practice of medicine, conducted through formal – very brief – encounters, has proved a key factor in the growing popularity of alternative practitioners, who offer more empathetic, more personal and lengthy consultations.

Over the past two decades a number of factors have encouraged orthodox doctors to take a greater interest in patients' attitudes towards health and illness. One is a lack of confidence in scientific medicine's capacity to deal with the prevalence of heart disease and cancer in an aging population. This has encouraged greater medical intervention in the patient's lifestyle aimed at preventing these diseases. Another is the paradox that, although objective indicators of health register steady improvement, people go to see doctors complaining of a wider range of physical symptoms, which are often inexplicable in terms of any recognised pathological process; they can be categorised as 'doing better, but feeling worse'. The dominant response to the problem of unexplained physical symptoms has been the expansion of the range of medical diagnosis and the re-labelling of collections of symptoms as new diseases, such as ME/chronic fatigue syndrome, repetitive strain injury, fibromyalgia and numerous psychiatric syndromes and disorders.

Unfortunately, medicine's turn towards the subjective has not been accompanied by a major expansion in the scientific study of what constitutes the experience of 'illness' or the interactions of the mind and the body in the genesis of symptoms. Earlier researches into the links between the nervous, endocrine and immune systems and their role in health and illness – in the new discipline dubbed psychoneuroimmunology in the 1980s – have been little developed in mainstream medicine; instead, it has been given a mystical interpretation and transformed into junk science by the practitioners of complementary therapies.

The shift of medicine away from the treatment of disease to the alleviation of the symptoms of illness in people in whom no disease process can be found has had important consequences. It has reinforced a trend towards the emergence of a society in which the state has sought to provide a range of therapeutic alternatives to orthodox medicine, including those of psychotherapy, counselling and complementary treatments. It legitimises the intrusion of the practice of medicine into the lifestyle of the individual and of society. Instead of these initiatives being 'as well as' they have become 'in place of' proper medicine. Today, modern doctors are expected to take on the tasks of social workers, teachers and the police, assuming a coercive role which can only prejudice the doctor–patient relationship.

Just as reason cannot co-exist with irrationality, so orthodox medicine cannot be reconciled with an alternative conflicting system. Astronomy and astrology are incompatible ways of studying the stars; alchemy and chemistry are fundamentally different concepts of the elements. Professor Ernst has described alternative medicine as 'a regressive temptation', 'the kind of medicine people took when there was no alternative'.

How can modern medicine begin to overcome its current predicament? It should stick to the rational principles that have made scientific medicine so successful in many spheres and establish a clear boundary between it and that of the non-rational belief systems with their non-scientific approach to healing. Doctors should resist the tendency to extend medical intervention into the wider areas of personal and social lifestyle and confine their efforts to their area of true expertise – the diagnosis and treatment of disease.

Research into the subjective aspects of illness and the effect of mental states on bodily function should be pursued scientifically. As the great nineteenth-century medical scientist Rudolph Virchow argued, 'One must learn and become accustomed to explain the unknown from the known, rather than the reverse.'

Chapter Thirty

EXERCISE AND SPORTS
BY PAUL AICHROTH

The Myth: **We should exercise as much as possible.**
The Fact: **Excessive exercise can cause more harm than good.**

The government exhorts us to take more exercise and play more sports, but how much exercise do we need? Preschool children hardly sit still for a moment until they collapse, exhausted, into sleep. Schoolchildren, on the other hand, sit at their desk all day, return home to confront their homework before seeking relaxation by flopping down in front of the television. It is this pattern of behaviour that they continue as adults when it becomes their established lifestyle. There are very good life-insurance statistics to show that a desk job and sedentary lifestyle is associated with a diminished life expectancy. This is a good reason to take exercise. The problem is, what type of exercise and how much? We hear of joggers dropping dead out running – indeed the president of the American Jogging Association did just that; youngish executives have suffered cardiac arrest playing squash; and many Olympic weightlifters, with their bulging muscles, run to seed, become fat and die prematurely.

If sport was innocent and health promoting, why would we need a medical speciality dealing with sports injury, and why are the orthopaedic wards of our hospitals filled by patients with sporting injuries and worn-out joints? Like any therapeutic activity, exercise should be prescribed in a suitable dose to meet specific indications. Against the backdrop of the overall advantage to those who take regular exercise, one must recognise that there are many situations in which a sport or exercise programme is unsuitable. One needs to get the subject into perspective, to understand where it may help and where it may be harmful.

EXERCISE AND THE HEART

The heart muscle, like that of any other muscle in the body, needs exercise if it is to be maintained in good condition. This is achieved every time one increases the amount of blood it pumps out, its cardiac output, in response to exertion or emotion. Like any pump, an increase in output can be achieved by pumping at a faster rate or by increasing the volume expelled during each cycle. Young people can easily increase the volume pumped, but this becomes increasingly restricted as one gets older. Older people respond to exercise by increasing the cardiac rate and the pulse rate. Unfortunately, increasing the heart rate actually diminishes the amount of blood and oxygen delivered to the heart muscle. As a result, in any person with diseased coronary blood vessels, the increased cardiac output required during exercise causes a reduction in blood flow to the heart at the very time it needs more oxygen. This produces angina. A sudden burst of excessive exercise in these patients will be dangerous. It is essential for any exercise regime in these patients to be monitored and carefully graded if a calamity is to be avoided.

EXERCISE AND OBESITY

Men who have been forced into prolonged, hard physical work without a compensatory increase in food intake, such as is the case with the survivors of labour camps, demonstrate the relationship between such work, calorie intake and weight. However, physical exercise, especially on a cold winter's day, stimulates the appetite; if there is free access to food, this will negate the anti-obesity effect. Regular exercise is believed to ratchet up the metabolic rate and it is this that will help keep the body weight in check.

It is largely through its effect on metabolic rate that exercise produces a loss of weight. The importance of the metabolic rate is demonstrated in patients in whom the metabolism is increased by disease, as is the case with thyrotoxicosis: in these patients, weight loss, in spite of a healthy appetite, is often a symptom. Occasional exercise, no mater how rigorous, is relatively less effective as a means of using up energy and producing a weight loss greater than regular activity would, as it is less likely to produce a prolonged increase in the metabolic rate. Most of the energy produced in the body goes towards maintaining body temperature; much less is used in muscle contraction. This effect is demonstrated by migrating birds that fly thousands of miles but seldom lose more than 15 per cent of their body mass.

EXERCISE AND DIABETES

Overweight patients who develop type-2 diabetes need to lose weight. Helmrich and his colleagues have shown that regular exercise will help to reduce the requirements of sugar-lowering drugs in these patients as well as helping them to lose weight.

EXERCISE AND THE MUSCLES

Physical strength depends upon us building up our muscles. One only has to observe the size of the muscles of the athlete, the village blacksmith or the weightlifter to appreciate the need for muscle bulk in this respect. The right limb of a right-handed individual is invariably stronger and larger than the left, as any tailor will tell you. The wasted limbs of the invalid who has been confined to bed is associated with considerable weakness when he tries to walk, a situation that requires appropriate training and exercise in order to correct it. In these patients, the skills of a good physiotherapist are essential to prescribe how best to strengthen the muscles without pain or damage. Left to their own, patients taking inappropriate exercise may actually delay their recovery.

The association between muscle power and increased muscle bulk produced by the use of steroids is less clear-cut. Although athletes taking these substances believe that their performance benefits, what little evidence there is suggests that, if this occurs, it only does so to a very limited extent.

One of the dangers of a sedentary individual suddenly adopting a vigorous exercise regime 'to get fit' or 'to lose weight', however, is that their muscles may have deteriorated and their tendons thinned to such an extent that they strain their muscles or rupture their tendons. Both of these painful conditions can take months to get better.

EXERCISE AND DAMAGED JOINTS

An acutely damaged joint will be swollen, stiff and painful. Such a joint should be rested. Exercising the joint will only aggravate the condition. The ideal treatment is to elevate the leg, rest it and apply an ice pack. Only when recovery starts to occur and the signs of inflammation disappear should a programme of exercise be started. This should aim to produce gentle, progressive muscle-strengthening.

Joints that have suffered longstanding damage will be much less inflamed and the pain associated with it may be reduced by movement and exercise in some patients. However, the puffy, swollen, painful joints associated with rheumatoid arthritis seldom benefit from exercise, and excessive exercise may be harmful. Osteoarthritis (better called osteoarthrosis) is a chronic degenerative condition associated with wear and tear of the joint surfaces. It is generally less painful than rheumatoid arthritis. In osteoarthritis it is important to keep the joint mobile and the surrounding muscles strong. Progressive, gentle stretching exercises, if possible under the weightless conditions of a hydrotherapy pool, are helpful. Good physiotherapists will often use local heat or ultrasound to help overcome muscle spasm and contraction. Without properly supervised exercise, this regime of 'fake, bake and ultraviolate', which is all that is offered in too many hospitals, is unlikely to be successful.

EXERCISE AND THE BRAIN

Two papers published in 2004 in the *Journal of the American Medical Association* have demonstrated that simply walking a few miles every day protects the elderly from mental decline and senile degeneration. They found that men between the ages of 71 and 93 who walked over two miles a mile a day had half the risk of senile dementia compared to those walking less than a quarter of a mile. A similar study in women confirmed that in women over 70 cognitive functions were better the further they walked. It could be argued that the group who walked furthest were self-selecting, as they were likely to have been more intelligent or more physically fit in the first place.

American figures suggest that more women than men become immobile as they grow older and that it is the men who are more likely to continue to take regular exercise over the age of 75. According to Bill Bryson (in *Made in America*), the average American walks as little as 1.2 miles a week, whereas it is recommended that this distance should be the minimum distance walked every day in order to protect one's health. It is little wonder that more Americans own walking machines, per capita, than anyone else.

Exercise has been shown to liberate endorphins, the natural opiate that causes a 'feel-good' factor. It is this that is responsible for the mood elevation, the 'high' that follows vigorous exercise. As a result it is advocated as a means of combating depression.

Regular exercise is said to increase the body's sensitivity to insulin and to combat some of the resistance to it that is a characteristic of type-2 diabetes.

SPORTS AND SPORTS INJURIES

Exercise and sports are really quite different things. Contact sports are enormously popular both with participants – who do the exercise and also receive the injuries – and those viewers who watch them sitting in a chair and doing no exercise at all. Most good players are fit, frequently superbly so. However, there is an inevitable price to pay by the very nature of the hard, physical contact involved. Broken bones, dislocated joints, torn ligaments and head injuries are not uncommon, especially at the weekends when large numbers are playing soccer, rugby, cricket or hockey. Horse riding, so popular in rural areas, has proved to be a dangerous pursuit. Accident and emergency departments in country areas are only too aware of the severe injuries that may occur to muscles, bones and to the spinal cord and skull from this form of exercise.

Common soccer and rugby injuries include rotational strains to knees causing torn cartilage and ruptured ligaments. Racing cyclists frequently suffer from the pain resulting from wearing out the lining of their kneecap. Gymnasts may place such sheering force on their joints that they rip the lining cartilage off the bone. Tennis players and ball throwers suffer from injuries to their shoulder joint and the capsule that surrounds it. Skiers damage their knees and their thumbs. Ten to twenty years ago they frequently broke the bones in their leg; today, with better-designed boots, it is commonly the knee ligaments that take the strain. Rollerbladers and snowboarders succumb to upper-limb injuries, especially affecting the wrist, shoulder and elbows.

In spite of this long list of injuries, some of which leave the participant in constant pain, some causing problems in later life and some ending fatally, we continue to encourage competitive sport and to regard it as a desirable form of exercise. In view of this, one would expect us to provide a service, similar to that available in the USA and continental Europe, for the treatment of sports injuries where the damage can be assessed and treated by specialist teams. In the UK, the NHS has all but ignored the need for these patients to receive immediate, high-calibre treatment. Instead, they have to wait their turn in many district hospitals while their problem becomes chronic and much more difficult to treat. This frequently results in long-term disability and a loss of that sportsman to his game.

JOGGING

Jogging is a popular form of exercise. It owes its popularity to the ease with which it may be carried out. All that is required is to put on a tracksuit and trainers and off one goes. Because the intensity of the exercise lies somewhere between running and walking, many jog in order to lose weight. Some people seem to be at ease jogging – watching them it appears to come naturally, and it is obviously a good form of exercise for them. Many, however, struggle and pound the ground in what appears to be a painful effort to jog; they probably should never have started. These joggers, generally overweight and with poor muscle tone, are likely to damage themselves by tearing muscles and straining ligaments. If they persist, they often wear out the linings of their joints and damage the cartilage in their knees. The force on the joints during jogging is enormous, especially if it is done inexpertly. Just walking downstairs exerts a force equal to four times one's body weight in the knee joint; if one runs upstairs, one may exert a force 15 times one's body weight. It is not surprising, therefore, to find knee problems in many of those who go jogging to lose weight or get fit.

WHAT EXERCISE IS NECESSARY?

Ideally one should take regular exercise, in the form of aerobic exercise and movement and stretching exercises, a few time every week.

The object of movement exercise is to achieve a full range of movement in all parts of the body, and stretching ensures the maintenance of the full extent of these functions. In addition to exercising all the major joints of the body – the hips, knees and shoulders – the various large groups of muscles controlling the joints such as the quadriceps muscles should be strengthened. Postural exercises to improve the way one stands and walks are valuable.

The simplest aerobic exercise is walking. Half an hour of brisk walking every day will provide sufficient aerobic exercise to offset any health disadvantage due to a sedentary lifestyle. If swimming or cycling are available, they are excellent additional forms of exercise.

Where a gym can be used, postural exercises and exercises to train the postural muscles will maintain muscle tone and counter some of the effects of age on one's sense of balance.

There is good evidence that the dangers of a sedentary existence justify the government's plea for us to take more exercise. There is *no* evidence that an excess of exercise or sports is of greater benefit to one's health than a brisk walk every day, although it may produce the added buzz of competition and the euphoria associated with the release of endorphins. Against this, however, should be weighed the very real risk of injury associated with many vigorous sports: unless they are expertly treated, many of these lead to permanent disabilities in later life. Sport is a double-edged sword: it can do harm as well good.

FURTHER READING

A LIST OF REFERENCES TO ARTICLES IN THE TEXT
IS HELD BY THE PUBLISHER

'Bamboozled, Baffled and Bombarded', Report of National
Consumer Council, 2002,
http://www.food.gov.uk/news/newsarchive/2003/feb/109303

'Clear Labelling Task Force', Food Standards Agency, 2002,
http://www.food.gov.uk/foodlabelling/researchandreports/49321

'Diet, Nutrition and preventing Chronic Disease', WHO, 2002,
http://www.who.int/hpr/NPH/docs/who_fao_expert_report.pdf

'Dietary Reference Values for Food Energy and Nutrients for the
United Kingdom: Report of the Panel on Dietary Reference Values
of the Committee on Medical Aspects of Food Policy',

'Dietary Value for food energy and Nutrition' HMSO, 1991

'Improving Children's Diet', Parliamentary Office of Science and
Technology, 2003, http://www.parliament.uk/post/pr199.pdf

Alderman, MH *et al*, 'Dietary Sodium Intake and Mortality: the National Health and Nutrition Examination Survey (NHANES I)', *The Lancet*, 351 (1998), pp 781-5

Andres, R, 'Mortality and Obesity: the rationale for age-specific height-weight tables': pp 311-318 in *Principles of Geriatric Medicine:* editors Andres R, Bierman, EL and Hazzard WR. (New York: McGraw-Hill Books, 1985)

Bunker, A, Houghton, J and Baum, M, 'Putting the risk of breast cancer in perspective', *BMJ*, 317 (1998), pp 1307-9.

Degregori, TR, *Origins of the Organic Agriculture Debate* (Blackwell Publishing, 2003)

Department of Health, 'Dietary Reference Values for Food Energy and Nutrients for the United Kingdom' (London: HMSO, 1991)

Dixon-Woods, M, 'Writing wrongs? An analysis of published discourses about the use of patient information leaflets' *Soc Sci Med* 52 (2001), pp 1417-32

Doll, K, Bradford Hill, A, 'Smoking and Carcinoma of the Lung', *BMJ* 30 September 1950, pp 740-9

Doll, R, Bradford Hill, A, 'Lung cancer and other causes of death in relation to smoking', *BMJ* 2 (1956), pp 1071-81

Doll, R, Bradford Hill, A, 'Mortality of doctors in relation to their smoking habits', *BMJ*, 26 June 1954, pp 1451-5

Fitzpatrick, M, *MMR and Autism: What Parents Need to Know* (London: Routledge, 2004)

Flechsig, E, Weissmann, C, 'The Role of PrP in Health and Disease' *Curr Mol Med* 4(4): pp 337-53

Furedi, F, 'The Politics of Fear', *spiked,* 28 October 2004, http://www.spiked-online.com/Printable/0000000CA760.htm

Glinsmann, W, Irausquin H, Park YK, 'Report from FDA's Sugars Task Force 1986: evaluation of health aspects of sugars contained in carbohydrate sweetners', *Journal of Nutrition*, 116 (November 1986), Supplement 118

Hackshaw, AK, Law, MR, Wald, NJ, 'The accumulated evidence on lung cancer and environmental tobacco smoke', *BMJ*, 315 (1997), pp 980-8

Horton, K, 'Screening mammography an overview revisited', *Lancet* 358 (2001), pp 1284-85

House of Lords Select Committee, 'Organic Farming and the European Union', 1999, Oral evidence, Q38

http://www.foodstandards.gov.uk/science

Huff, D, *How to Lie with Statistics*, (Pelican Books, 1954)

Humphrey, LL, Helfand M, Benjamin KS, Chan MS, Woolf SH, 'Breast Cancer Screening: A Summary of the Evidence for the US Preventive Services Task Force', *Annals of Internal Medicine* 137 (2002), pp 347-60.

Institute of Medicine, 'Dietary Reference Intakes for Vitamin A, Vitamin K, Arsenic, Boron, Chromium, Copper, Iodine, Iron,

Manganese, Molybdenum, Nickel, Silicon, Vanadium and Zinc' (Washington DC: National Academy Press, 2000)

Institute of Medicine, 'Dietary Reference Values for Vitamin C, Vitamin E, Selenium and Carotenoids', (Washington DC: National Academy Press, 2000), http://www.iom.edu/report.asp?id=8511

Klatsky, AL, 'Drink to your Health', *Scientific American*, 283 (Feb 2003), p 62-9

Lachmann, PJ, 'Diet and Diseases: Facts and Fantasies', 1999, http://www.acmedsci.ac.uk/n_diet.htm

Maddox, J, *The Doomsday Syndrome*, (Macmillan 1972), p 110

Moore, P. 'Environmentalism for the 21st century', www.greenspirit.com

NHS Centre for Reviews and Dissemination, 'Report 18. A Systematic Review of Water Fluoridation', September 2000, http://www.york.ac.uk/inst/crd/pdf/fluorid.pdf

Nuffield Council on Bio-ethics, GM Crops in Developing Countries, January, 2004, p 53

Nuffield, 'GM crops: ethical and social issues', 1999, http://www.nuffieldbioethics.org/go/ourwork/gmcrops/publication_301.html

Pastana, C, *Fluids and Electrolytes* (Baltimore: Williams & Wilkins 1980)

Rayman, M, 'The importance of selenium to human health', *Lancet,* 356 (2000), pp 233-41

Reichman, WJ, *Use and Abuse of Statistics* (Penguin Books, 1952)

Royal Society *et al*, 'Transgenic Plants and World Agriculture', July 2000 http://www.agbios.com/docroot/articles/2000192-A.pdf

Report on Health and Social Subjects, 41 (London: HMSO, 1991)

Schlosser, E, *Fast Food Nation* (Penguin Books, 2001)

Skrabanek, P, 'Mass mammography. The time for reappraisal', *Int J Technol Assess Health Care*, 5 (1989), pp 423-30.

The GM Science Review, 2003/2004, http://www.gmsciencedebate.org.uk/

The Royal Society, 'GMOs and Pusztai', 1999

Various authors, 'New Approaches to define Nutrient Requirements', *American Journal of Clinical Nutrition,* 63 (1996), pp 983-1001

Verney, EB, 'Renal Excretion of Water and Salt', *Lancet* 1237 (1957)

Will, R, 'Variant Creutzfeldt-Jakob disease' *Folia Neuropathol* 42 Suppl A, (2004) 77–83.

Willett, WC & Stampfer, MJ, 'Rebuilding the Food Pyramid' *Scientific American* 2003: 298 (Jan):52-59